Eagletree Herbs Guide

to Herbal Medicine Making

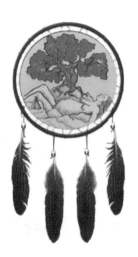

Eagletree Herbs Guide to Medicine Making

Daphne Singingtree

ISBN: 978-0-9674431-6-4

1st Edition July 2024

Book Cover *Mary Glor Cuda*

Editing *Lili Booth*

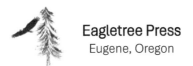

Eagletree Press
Eugene, Oregon

www.eagletreepress.com

Dedicated to my children, Alder, Aradia, Terran and Trillium, who grew up working in the herbal business, whether they liked it or not.

Also dedicated to all the students, interns and helpers I have over the years who inspired and encouraged me, as well as gave invaluable practical help. I could not have done it without you.

Contents

Body Care

Body Care: Facial

Body Care: Men's Line

Culinary Superfoods 114

Salts & Superfood Seasonings

Syrups–Culinary

Vinegars

First Aid

Love Products

Maternity and Baby

Pest Control

Salves and Balms

Smoking Blends

Syrups & Elixirs—Medicinal

Teas

Afterwards 160

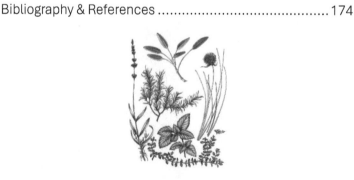

Chapter One
Journey Begins

How I Became an Herbal Medicine Maker

Herbal medicine saved my life. I'm not saying I had a life-threatening disease and herbs miraculously cured me, although that happens sometimes to some individuals. It was the study of herbs and holistic medicine that changed the entire trajectory of my life, which could have gone in a very different and dangerous direction.

I left home and began living on my own when I was twelve years old. Not exactly left home, as my family was homeless. I was not a runaway, as my mother never reported me missing to the police. She assumed I could take care of myself. It sounds terrible from a modern standpoint, but it was 1970. The hippie movement had just begun, and life was very different. There were many teenage runaways. I looked older and knew how to take care of myself.

Drugs were a part of street life, and I started down that road. I had a bad acid trip and ended up in police custody. My parents divorced when I was four years old, resulting in losing contact with my dad. The authorities tracked down my adult sister. Both she and my grandmother had long been estranged from my mother. I had not seen either of them since I was a small child. I went to live with them in Red Bluff, California. Living with my sister, her husband, children, and my grandmother was the first time in my life where I had stability. It was everything I had always thought I wanted: a "normal" middle-class life. There was no drama, no abuse, enough food, and the utilities were never turned off. Prior to this, I had attended sixteen different elementary schools before leaving in the sixth grade. In Red Bluff, I went back to school. My sister even had a horse that I learned to ride. They were wonderful to me, but I was bored stiff. I lasted a couple of months living with my sister and grandmother. After living on my own for so long, living a "normal" life was not for me.

I met some hitchhikers who told me about Rainbow Farm, a commune open to anyone. The next day, I left and hitchhiked to Rainbow Farm. There I was introduced to the book *Back to Eden* by Jethro Kloss. It changed my life; it became my bible. *The Herbalist* by John Meyer was another early herb book I treasured. I discovered home birth, organic gardening, and a lifestyle that would later be termed "off grid." Embracing a holistic lifestyle kept me away from a dark path many young girls in my situation ended up on.

I attended the first Rainbow Gathering in 1972 and from there I traveled, working various jobs that required the fake ID I got, claiming I was eighteen. I hitchhiked all over the country with a heavy backpack full of herb books and little glass jars full of dried herbs. Not sure why I didn't have them in plastic bags. While living in Berkeley, California, I found some wonderful herb classes taught by an older naturopathic doctor, Mildred Jackson, who wrote *The Handbook to Alternatives to Chemical Medicine*. I still remember her remedy for bladder infections: take a full bulb of garlic, crush slightly, put in a quart jar, cover the garlic with boiling water, cover, let sit until cool, then fill half the jar with water and drink the whole thing before bed, so the garlic will stay in your bladder as long as possible.

My parents divorced when I was four years old, and I never saw my father again. I had known my father was part Lakota, but I did not know which tribe, nor did I know anything about my Native heritage. When I turned fifteen, in honor of that heritage, I changed my name to Singingtree, seeking that connection. It was not until I was in my fifties that one of my aunts found me online, told me they had been looking for me for years to let me know I inherited land on the Standing Rock Reservation, as my father had passed away some years before.

I wish I had connected with my father's family earlier and could study from my tribe's elders. By studying on my own, learning from whoever I could, and dosing myself and everyone I knew with various herbal teas, I gradually became knowledgeable enough to share what I knew. I started teaching herb classes when I was fifteen. In 1973, after teaching a class at the Whole Earth Festival in Davis, California, I met the man who would later become my husband and the father of my first child. Russell Nickels called Rusty back then. He is a medical doctor trained in pediatrics and later certified in family medicine. He was also a speaker at the festival and was giving a presentation and showing a film about home birth. The film was so moving and powerful it started me on the road to becoming a midwife. The presenter, Rusty, was amazing, and I fell madly in love with him. He had long braids down to his back, a hippie doctor who believed in herbs and home birth. Although he did not have tribal heritage, he had a deep respect for Indigenous medicine, which he studied.

He was thirty-four, and I was fifteen. In today's world, he would face arrest, despite the fact that our relationship was not only consensual, but I relentlessly pursued him all over the country. Back then, it may have been uncommon, but was not all that unusual. It was a different time and a different culture.

He taught me so much. I attended home births with him, my apprenticeship in midwifery. He founded a nonprofit organization called the Tribal Healing Council. He had a grant to study natural alternatives to drug abuse, so we traveled all over, attended a lot of sweat lodges and peyote meetings, and visited reservations to learn about natural medicine. We traveled to Mexico and went to Guatemala, where he taught and I became a student at *Instituto Naturista*, a natural healing school run by the Seventh Day Adventists to train medical missionaries. I had my 16th birthday in Guatemala. It was an extraordinary experience. We talked to Indigenous healers wherever we went.

When I was seventeen, we got married and planned to conceive our son Alder, who was born when I was eighteen. We only stayed together for a few years after that because somehow, I thought there were perfect men out there. He was not only the love of my life, but an important teacher in both midwifery and medicine.

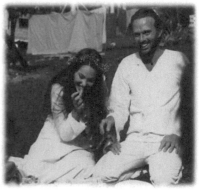

Daphne and Rusty Wedding 1975

The Oregon Country Fair (OCF)

In 1974, I began attending the Oregon Country Fair (OCF), a large art and music festival held annually in July near Veneta, Oregon. OCF, a nonprofit organization, owns and maintains the land where the festival is held, and vendors keep their booths year-round.

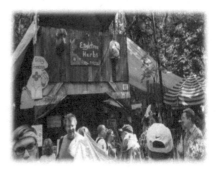

2006 Booth at OCF

It's a massive event requiring thousands of volunteers and has cultivated its own distinctive culture. My entry into the business of herbal products began with vending at the Oregon Country Fair. In the initial years, I taught herb classes from my tipi. By the time my son was nearly two, we secured the booth where we still vend today.

I was focused on practicing midwifery, and our booth served as an information hub for midwifery. I crafted a few herbal remedies, particularly those related to pregnancy.

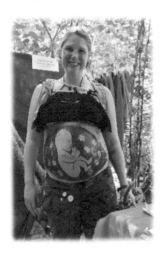

Belly painted mama 2023

On our first night there, mosquitoes swarmed, leaving my young son covered in bites. After returning home, I concocted a batch of herbal mosquito repellent to sell. It contained a base of sunflower oil with essential oils of camphor for soothing bites, along with citronella, eucalyptus, pennyroyal, and a touch of cinnamon. The repellent, later named Mosquidaddle, proved immensely popular. That first year, I had to mix batches right in the back of the booth. For many years, the sales from Mosquidaddle covered all our booth expenses while we promoted midwifery, painted pregnant women's bellies, and expanded our herbal product offerings each year. We had some hits and misses. Some products everyone loved, others sat on the shelf for years. Never did market research, which is a key to successful businesses. Guesses are not the same.

My four children grew up helping. While they complained as they grew older, they loved it too. There is so much work involved, not only in making all the products, but camping at a large festival. All my kids grew up to be very hard workers, and I attribute some of that to the Oregon Country Fair.

My youngest daughter, Trillium, is the most involved. She is now the one that paints the pregnant women's bellies. Many of the products are her creations, especially the ones with cute names. She is now taking over the booth; the herbs are gradually going away. Outside of their electrician jobs, she sews and designs amazing clothing and with her husband they make cool leather top hats.

How Eagletree Herbs Began

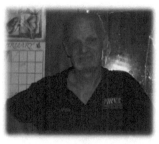

Michael Eagle 1944-2013.

In the 1980s, I met Michael Eagle, who became my best friend and business partner. Combining elements of both our names, we christened our venture Eagletree Herbs, also adopting the name for my publishing business, Eagletree Press, which until then only published my midwifery books. Sadly, in 2013, Michael passed away; you can read more about his life on the Eagletree Herbs website. In 2002, after thirty years of practicing and teaching midwifery, I retired to focus entirely on Eagletree Herbs.

Over time, we expanded our offerings to include culinary and body care products, with tinctures, over 100 different products. I converted my suburban front lawn to cultivate herbs. We converted my former laundry room into a small commercial kitchen and distributed products through local stores. We vended at many events, such as farmer's markets and local festivals.

For years, I ran an intern program where four to six interns would join us twice a week for three months to help grow and make products. Each week, they presented herb reports, sharing their newfound knowledge with the group.

I loved making new products; I am sure I would have been more successful as a business with more focus and fewer products. People would come up to our booth at an event and ask if we had an herbal product that we did not make, and I thought sure that is easy, and would make it to have at the next event.

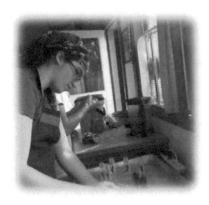
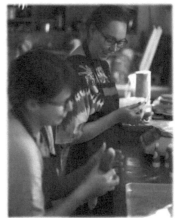
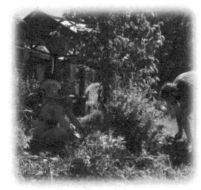
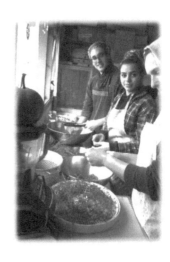
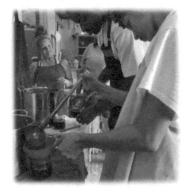

I never would have been able to run the business without the interns. They helped in the garden, harvest and prepared the herbs, helped make the products, and helped sell them by vending at events.

My Struggle with Obesity

Over the years, I gradually gained weight until I became morbidly obese, severely affecting my ability to function. Despite my extensive knowledge of nutrition and holistic health, I was dismayed at how I had allowed myself to reach this state. My morbid obesity, a complex condition with both mental and physiological factors, proved resistant to many diets I attempted over the years, including vegan, paleo, keto, and intermittent fasting. Each time, I would lose a little weight, only to regain it—and more—in a vicious cycle known as yo-yo dieting. As my weight increased, exercise became difficult, leading to a more sedentary lifestyle. Unfortunately, the more sedentary you are, the more sedentary you become.

I started an online midwifery school and spent years working at the computer ten to twelve hours every day. When I wasn't seated at the computer, I was in front of the TV or in my recliner with a book. My weight ballooned to the point where I could no longer fit behind the wheel of my car, and I developed numerous weight-related health problems.

After extensive research, surgery seemed like the only viable option for someone of my size to lose weight. Despite my lifelong aversion to unnecessary surgeries, I opted for weight loss surgery in 2011 as a last resort. I chose a vertical gastric sleeve, a newer and less invasive procedure that reduces stomach size without bypassing the stomach and small intestine.

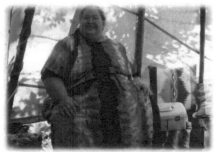

Hard to believe I got this big. In my tipi, OCF 2010.

To qualify for surgery, I had to lose forty pounds, which became a powerful motivator. Rather than attempting another diet, I took up gardening, which allowed me to engage in physical activity at a manageable pace. Using a calorie counting app proved beneficial. After about six months, I successfully lost enough weight to qualify for the surgery.

The surgery was successful initially, and I lost nearly 100 pounds. My quality of life improved significantly—I gained a new boyfriend, had more energy, and felt optimistic about the future. However, I began experiencing issues with low blood pressure post-surgery, which seemed manageable at first.

Car Accident

While driving, my blood pressure suddenly dropped, causing me to pass out and veer across two lanes of the Northwest Expressway before crashing into a bridge. The accident resulted in severe injuries to both of my legs. One leg sustained a compound fracture (bone protruding), while the other leg suffered three fractures along with broken ankles. Thanks to a gifted orthopedic surgeon, my legs were reconstructed using extensive hardware. Given my weight, diabetes, and surgical wounds, the risk of infection and potential amputation of one or both legs were alarmingly high. It remained uncertain whether I would regain the ability to walk.

Following the hospitalization, I was in a nursing home; it was horrible. Fortunately, my boyfriend took proactive measures, building a ramp and installing grab bars at home. We arranged for a hospital bed and secured full-time home health aides, allowing me to transition back home from the nursing facility. I was never so happy to be home.

I drank a lot of comfrey and horsetail tea because of their bone healing properties. We made kombucha with white tea and nettles to prevent infections. I strongly believe these treatments contributed significantly to my recovery, as I avoided infections and gradually my bones healed.

Although I have regained some mobility, it remains limited, and much of the weight has returned, leaving me still battling obesity. I am still about 100 lbs. less than my highest weight but still need to lose about 100 more. I can walk now, relying on a combination of walker and canes for support, although I need a wheelchair for longer distances. Despite these challenges, I am managing reasonably well, though I still require help with certain tasks.

Gardening is something I can manage with help, as I can sit down often and pace myself. Learning permaculture has been rewarding, and between housemates and home helpers we have a been able to have a small urban homestead.

The Kale Sprinkles Story

Struggling with arthritis following the accident, I sought herbs to alleviate the inflammation. Alongside my arthritis tincture, I developed Kale Sprinkles, a seasoning blend incorporating foods and herbs known for their anti-inflammatory properties (recipe page 112). It quickly became one of our most popular and profitable products. We had fun marketing it; our interns dressed as "Kale Fairies"

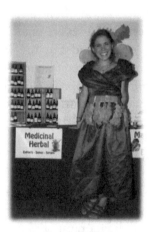

Sara as Kale Fairy

in green costumes with fairy wings, and adorned with live kale leaves, distributing free samples at events and stores.

Kale Sprinkles had so much potential we found an investor. We thought after all these years we were turning the corner, from being a hobby to a sustainable business. We hired more staff, got in more stores, and were on the way to becoming profitable.

Then I left for several months because of Standing Rock and had very little internet access. The phones were unreliable, and I did not call in often, leaving the business in the hands of part-time employees. They were wonderful and supportive, but it was not the same. As any entrepreneur knows, one needs to focus and work hard to make any business successful.

When I returned, things had changed. Primarily was my desire to focus more on herbs and less on the business side of things.

The Standing Rock Protests

In 2016, the Dakota Access Pipeline (DAPL) planned to install an oil pipeline under the river that supplied the Standing Rock Sioux Reservation's drinking water, despite strong objections from the tribe. Given the frequent leaks in pipelines, the project posed a significant threat to the water supply and the surrounding ecosystem. Tribal citizens and their allies established a camp along the pipeline's proposed route to protest and raise awareness.

The protest camp initially comprised a few dozen youth activists, women, and local residents, but quickly grew into a

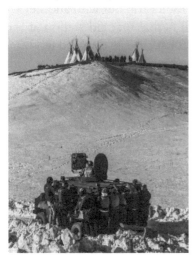

massive gathering supported by volunteers and donations from around the world—all united to safeguard the water. It marked the largest assembly of Native American tribes in history. People from all over the world came and took part,

Military style police at Standing Rock Protests

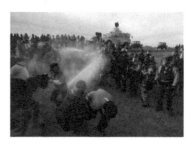

and it was devoid of formal leadership or centralized organization.

Only a few years earlier, I had connected with my father's family and discovered I had inherited fractionated land on the Standing Rock Reservation, jointly owned and leased. I felt deeply connected to the Standing Rock reservation, although I never owned a piece of land I could stand on. Monitoring the protests closely through social media, I raised funds and sent donations. Witnessing livestreams of protestors being injured compelled me to act. My niece Leah joined me, and we drove to South Dakota with a U-Haul packed with herbs and supplies to establish a free tea station. Once set up, we provided a place to distribute the herbal donations pouring in.

It was profoundly moving and empowering to give away herbs and medicines. I learned from the Native people about their herbal traditions, aided by resources like *Native American Ethnobotany* by Daniel E. Moerman to translate names of herbs from their native languages to the English or Latin name of the plant. The experience enriched my soul in a way that learning about herbs from books or classes never did.

Upon returning home, I made another trip out with another U-Haul of donations, setting up an herbal first aid station at the Rosebud camp across the river. A generously donated tipi bore my logo, which we designated an herb tipi. We sorted through

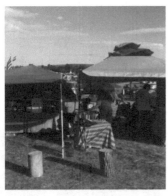

Tea station main camp August 2016

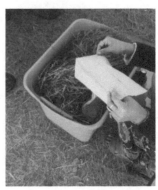

I brought totes of lavender to give away

countless boxes, distributing herbs and preparing large batches of tea. Gallons of fire cider and elderberry syrup were served. Working with the many volunteers, including the doctors who traveled from afar to support the Water Protectors and oppose DAPL, was humbling.

While DAPL ultimately succeeded in installing the pipeline beneath the reservation's water supply, the broader struggle to safeguard water and protect the earth had only just begun.

The legacy of Standing Rock continues to influence corporate practices, compelling closer adherence to environmental protections, if for no other reason, to avoid a massive protest and PR nightmare.

Personally, the experience transformed me. Giving away medicine instead of selling it felt liberating, prompting a gradual shift in priorities. After several years, I am now retiring from business, gradually selling off back stock, and vending solely in the Oregon Country Fair. This herbal guide is a way to pass on my knowledge, recipes, and experiences in fifty years of medicine making. I am focusing my energies on writing and just completed my debut speculative fiction novel, *Circle for the Earth A Time Travel Saga for a Sustainable Future.* I hope to spend more time on the Standing Rock Reservation in the future, as I made some wonderful connections at my time in the protest camps.

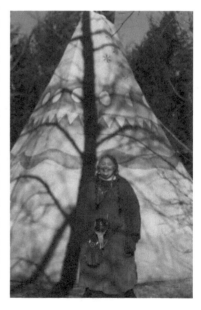

Daphne in front of her tipi at Rosebud camp

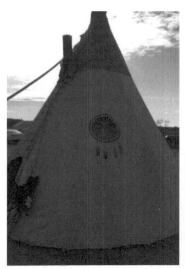
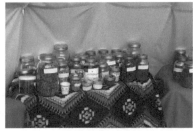
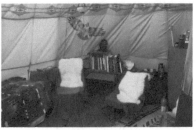

My herbal tipi at the Rosebud camp

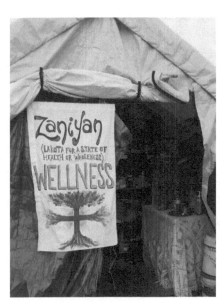
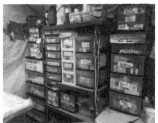
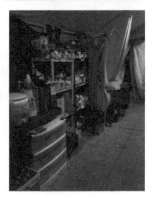

Herbal first aid station Rosebud Camp

Chapter Two
Getting Started

Healing Our Relationship with Plants

The word for plants in some Indigenous languages means *Those who take care of us.* We now consume and use many plants that are made available through methods and practices that lack integrity and are harmful to the planet. We may also be guilty of mindless consumption without a spiritual foundation in our use of plants. It is important to acknowledge the value in all ancestral teachings & traditions, including African, Asian, Celtic, European, Mideastern, Indigenous, and Wise Woman.

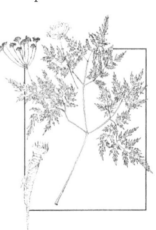

Knowing each specific plant, listening to its spirit or qualities, like the best season to harvest, or which part to harvest, respects the plant's individual and unique essence.

Osha root, also called Bear Root

Names have power. Plant names differ between common, Latin, and all the different languages used. Learning the names can help you connect to the plant. Sometimes the name of the plant reflects its usage, like lungwort.

Questions to ask. Did your ancestors use this plant? How do various traditions around the world use this plant? What areas is the plant native to? How did it migrate to where it grows now?

Listening to plants involves paying attention to how and where they grow. What does the plant need from us to be healthy? Learn from others about protocols the plant requires for healthy and balanced collection and use?

Check if a plant is **endangered** or **over-harvested** before you go wildcrafting. Never take more than you need for one season, and only take about one fourth of the plant unless specially grown.

United Plant Savers is a nonprofit organization working to prevent the loss of these important plants. They publish lists of endangered medicinal herbs.

Endangered Plant List 2024:

"CRITICAL"

- **Elephant Tree** – _Bursera microphylla_
- **False Unicorn** – _Chamaelirium luteum_
- **Lady's Slipper Orchid** – _Cypripedium_ spp.
- **Peyote** – _Lophophora williamsii_
- **Sandalwood** – _Santalum_ spp. (Hawaii only)
- **Sundew** – _Drosera_ spp.
- **Trillium, Beth Root** – _Trillium_ spp.
- **Venus Fly Trap** – _Dionaea muscipula_

"AT-RISK"

- **American Ginseng** – _Panax quinquefolius_
- **Black Cohosh** – _Actaea racemosa_
- **Bloodroot** – _Sanguinaria canadensis_
- **Blue Cohosh** – _Caulophyllum thalictroides_
- **Butterfly Weed** – _Asclepias tuberosa_
- **Cascara Sagrada** – _Frangula purshiana_
- **Chaparro** – _Castela emoryi_
- **Echinacea** – _Echinacea_ spp.
- **Gentian** – _Gentiana_ spp.
- **Goldenseal** – _Hydrastis canadensis_
- **Goldthread** – _Coptis_ spp.

- **Kava** – *Piper methysticum* (Hawaii only)
- **Lomatium** – *Lomatium dissectum*
- **Maidenhair Fern** – *Adiantum pedatum*
- **Mayapple** – *Podophyllum peltatum*
- Oregon Root – *Berberis* spp.
- **Osha** – *Ligusticum porteri*
- Partridge Berry – *Mitchella repens*
- **Pink Root** – *Spigelia marilandica*
- **Pipsissewa** – *Chimaphila umbellata*
- **Ramps** – *Allium tricoccum*
- **Slippery Elm** – *Ulmus rubra*
- **Squirrel Corn** – *Dicentra canadensis*
- **Stone Root** – *Collinsonia canadensis*
- **Stream Orchid** – *Epipactis gigantea*
- **True Unicorn** – *Aletris farinosa*
- **Virginia Snakeroot** – *Aristolochia serpentaria*
- **White Sage** – *Salvia apiana*
- **Wild Indigo** – *Baptisia tinctoria*
- **Wild Yam** – *Dioscorea villosa*
- **Yerba Mansa** – *Anemopsis californica*

"IN REVIEW"

- **Arnica** – *Arnica* spp.
- Chaga – *Inonotus obliquus*
- **Eyebright** – *Euphrasia* spp.
- Ghost Pipe – *Monotropa uniflora*
- **Lobelia** – *Lobelia inflata*
- Skunk Cabbage – *Symplocarpus foetidus*
- Solomon's Seal – *Polygonatum biflorum*
- Wild Cherry – Prunus serótina

Using Plants for Medicine

When you first start learning about herbs, it's tempting to focus on memorizing which plant treats which condition. With so many herbs offering diverse benefits, the sheer volume of information can quickly become overwhelming. Quality and depth matter more than sheer quantity when studying herbs. Emphasize evidence-based research and personal experience with each plant. Beyond reading, actively use herbs to experience their effects on your body. Grow or wild-harvest them, dry and prepare them in various ways—raw, in teas, tinctures, or for external applications. Apprentice yourself to the plant. Master one plant thoroughly before moving to others. Take the initiative to identify the plants that grow around you or are easily obtained and learn all the properties they   offer.

Learn botany. There are wonderful books, and all kinds of free resources on the internet. Knowledge is power. Learning botany basics will help you in plant identification and give you wonderful tools.

It is surprising how few herbs can treat a wide variety of conditions. There is so much to know about herbs and so many

Principal Parts of a Vascular Plant

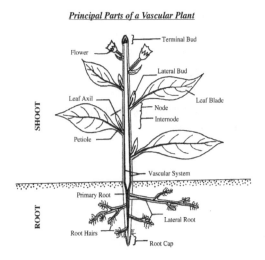

herbalists with lifetimes of knowledge and experience to share. Books and the internet offer valuable information, yet some sources may be inaccurate, misleading, or contradictory. Critically evaluate sources by checking if they aim to sell products or attract clicks.

Verify information's reproducibility across multiple reliable sources. Does it provide references on where the information came from? Wikipedia is an excellent resource for checking medicinal uses of plants because it provides links to scientific studies. If you are doing an internet search on the medicinal properties of a specific plant, use Google Scholar to eliminate clickbait and get clinical studies or historical uses.

Research On Herbs Can Be Flawed

As plant actions can vary on different animals, not all animal studies can or should be extrapolated to humans. Many reports isolated in vitro (outside of the body) study results without consideration of actual in vivo (inside the body) experience. Thus, some herbs may be harmful or helpful based on theoretical concerns that have not been proven in vivo. Drug or supplement companies pay for research, they have a profit motive, and their results may affect that agenda.

Judging an herb by individual constituents does not consider the possibly ameliorating effects of its other constituents. Herbs work synergistically, in harmony, with many constituents not yet identified by science. Spiritual aspects of the plant, including the intention of its harvest and preparation, is not something that can be quantified and measured. Nature holds mystery.

While herbalists are not doctors, they are health educators. If you are recommending herbal medicines, it's crucial to have basic health knowledge. While knowing twenty herbs for respiratory conditions is valuable, understanding the distinctions between illnesses like bronchitis and pneumonia, or recognizing when a fever may be life-threatening, is essential. This kind of knowledge is simple and easy to get. Right next to your herb books should be some health books, like *Where There Is No Doctor* by the Hesperian Foundation. There are community health worker programs, some available for free and online.

Dr. Google can be helpful when learning about various health conditions. Knowing the signs and symptoms of various conditions, and what conditions may mimic other conditions (differential diagnosis) are as important as knowing which herb is good for what. Knowing your limitations and when to refer someone to additional health knowledge is critical.

Plants are amazing at healing. Properly growing, harvesting, and preparing herbs can turn them into powerful medicine. They can sometimes be more effective than conventional medicine and often complement medical treatments. Modern medicine excels in diagnosis, backed by extensive training. Nature is healing, yet can be harsh; historically, high infant mortality meant only the strongest survived.

Many turn to herbs and holistic medicine because of negative experiences with the medical system or a desire to avoid conventional treatments. When looking at how the medical insurance industrial complex, pharmaceutical companies, and how current medical systems can fail individuals, it is understandable.

In our eagerness to explore alternative approaches, we should be cautious not to completely reject conventional medicine. While criticisms of the medical establishment are valid, integrating knowledge from various sources—including conventional medicine—can optimize health outcomes. Using knowledge and tools from various sources can make a difference. Gather information and knowledge from as many places as you can, look at the individual, and plan to use the medicine that will work best.

A lesson I learned from midwifery was to use Evidence-Based medicine, which is a systematic approach that uses scientific evidence to help make decisions about care. It's a lifelong process that involves integrating clinical expertise with research evidence and patient values. While used in medical care, it is important in holistic care as well, to look at science although it is only one aspect.

Learning to use plants for medicine is more than the physical, but a spiritual, mental, and emotional process. When you grow and wildcraft plants for medicine with the intention of healing you bring in a part of yourself. When you share that medicine with those you care about, you give them a bit of your energy and your love. Plants have their own spirit, their own energy, they give their life to you, and that medicine when acknowledged can be powerful.

When can using herbs be harmful?

- If the plant is not properly identified.
- If the dosage is used incorrectly.
- If the preparation was improper, such as being unsanitary or using unsafe canning practices.
- With an allergic reaction or sensitivity to a specific herb.
- If an interaction occurs between an herb and a prescribed medication.
- Improper harvesting, storing, or processing of the plant usually renders it ineffective rather than harmful.
- If someone neglects illness, if the herbs are not working after a reasonable period and someone avoids seeking medical attention.
- Taken in pill form changes and concentrates constituents.
- If contaminated with chemicals or other harmful substances.
- If the wrong part of the plant is used.
- Occasionally during pregnancy & breastfeeding.

Herbs Are Not Drugs, or Are They?

- Standardizing and put into pill form puts herbs on the road to being drugs.
- Standardizing is useful for research, which can be important in determining safety.
- While there is some regulation of herbs, quality/potency can vary quite a bit, especially with standardized vs. non-standardized.
- A standardized herbal extract has one or more components present in a specific, guaranteed amount, usually expressed as a percentage.
- Some herbs marketed as supplements, prescribed by some naturopathic doctors, and/or regulated by the FDA, are usually standardized.
- Companies often standardize herbs when they sell them as capsules, extracts, or concentrates.
- When put into pill form, it concentrates the herbs which change and concentrate constituents not found in nature.

Plants Teach Us

- They are whole, complex, and comprise parts that can't be separated like drugs.
- Can be nourishing, strengthening, and supportive of healing.
- Plants grown, wildcrafted, harvested, and processed as intentionally as medicine have intrinsic value not recognized by science.
- As each person has unique health needs, plants are also unique. What herbs work for one person may not work for another.
- Plants support the body to heal itself.
- Using plants for medicine connects us to the earth. The earth brings healing.

The Business of Eagletree Herbs

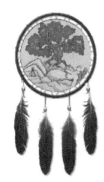

While Eagletree Herbs was never profitable, during busy years, we supported three to five part-time staff. Transitioning from a family enterprise to employing staff and navigating taxes, regulations, insurance, and licensing presented challenges.

In the earliest days, my children helped a great deal, especially helping vend at events. When they were little, they were so cute hawking mosquito repellent, offering free samples and rattling off the ingredients. When they grew up, my daughter Trillium continued to help, and developed many of our best-selling products.

In any business, you need to look at the cost of goods and the cost of labor to set your prices. I was never very good at that, choosing organic, when conventional was less expensive. We had an advantage with the intern program helping with production and keeping labor costs down. Applying business principles was never my forte, and it showed. I was not very good at things like tracking inventory.

Like any small business, marketing was crucial, yet I lacked the enthusiasm to dedicate time to it. Fortunately, many customers who saw us at the Oregon Country Fair and other events continued to reorder from our website. Gradually, we downsized to a single part-time employee and maintained a barely break-even status for years. It was more of a passion project than a profitable venture. However, it allowed me to work outdoors, cultivate herbs, interact with interns, teach, and create herbal remedies. It allowed me to have medicines to give away and barter, which I love. The work itself was its own reward.

Tips for Growing an Herbal Business

Learn from my mistakes and things I wish I knew beforehand:

- Start with a realistic business plan.
- Honestly assess the time commitment needed, then double it—everything takes longer than expected.
- If lacking business experience, seek guidance from friends, family, or community resources.
- Budget for materials, labor, and your own time.
- Differentiate your products to minimize competition.
- Begin small and simple, focus on a few unique products you do well.
- Grow as many of your herbs as possible.
- Leverage social media as your primary marketing tool.
- Network with herbalists, health practitioners, and potential collaborators.
- Expand beyond online to community events, farmers' markets, and local stores.
- Host workshops or speak at community events to educate people about herbs.
- Have a mechanism for getting feedback and reviews for your products.
- Focus on what sells well. If it doesn't sell, drop.
- Stay updated with the latest research and trends in herbal medicine and business practices.
- Keep a good inventory of containers and ingredients you use to make products. Only buy what you need.
- Join online support groups of other herbal entrepreneurs.
- Make educational video shorts for social media about specific herbs.
- Love, love, herbs, and let it show.

Create A Business Plan

There are lots of free online resources available online as well as your local small business associations. Use all the traditional business help you can find.

Analyze Your Business Using SWOT

Strengths, Weaknesses, Opportunities and Threats

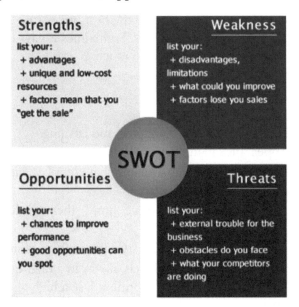

Have an Effective Online Presence

- Pay an established web hosting company like Wix or GoDaddy. They are reliable and integrate your payments. They have easy-to-use templates and require no web experience.
- If you don't want pay a large monthly fee, and don't mind a learning curve, use WordPress.
- Use Etsy or similar online marketplaces.
- Research SEO to add to your site.
- Share links with other sites whenever you can.
- Write a blog. Use Tiktok and Instagram.

Source Your Materials

- Identify reputable and ethical vendors for materials you can't grow, such as Mountain Rose Herbs.
- Consider vendors offering credit options for established businesses.
- Find wildcrafters in your area if you cannot do it yourself.
- Spend time online finding the best prices for containers and ingredients. Sometimes it pays to buy in bulk, other times not so much.

Packaging & Labeling

- Develop attractive packaging and labeling. Appearance matters.
- Create informative packaging that complies with regulatory requirements.
- Take the time to observe how other products are packaged.
- Develop your own brand style that reflects your values.
- If you print your own labels, invest in a high-quality laser, **not** an inkjet color printer. Use a high gloss label.
- Avery.com has a free online program for labels. No need for a graphic designer, very easy to use.
- Make sure everything is sparkling clean. If you attend a lot of outdoor events with a lot of dust, stay away from white or light colors.
- Implement Lot Numbers: For instance, use the format year-batch number (e.g., 2024-2 for the second batch in 2024). This system helps easily identify the age of products from their labels.
- Come up with catchy and fun names for products.

What Information to Include When Labeling
(from Mountain Rose Herbs)

Labels should include as much information as possible. It helps keep track of the ingredients and the age of the product, but it is also vital information for the next time we use those ingredients. These details make it easier to re-create a recipe or to tinker with it to achieve better results. Which details to include on your label depends on what you are making, but some important items include:

- Common name (essential for identification purposes)
- Latin name (optional, but often recommended because different plants can share common names, whereas the Latin name is always a distinct identifier)
- Plant part used (essential for safety considerations)
- Fresh/Dried (optional, but recommended to help you formulate the same recipe again)
- The ratio of herb to liquid menstruum—ie:1:2 or 1:5 (essential for dosage considerations and formulating the same blend in the future)
- Alcohol% (essential when using alcohol as the menstruum)
- Habitat/Source (optional, but if you are wild harvesting, a note like "Coniferous woods, 2,000 feet elevation" can be useful)
- Date formulation made (essential to keep track of shelf life and next steps like straining)
- Dosage (optional, but recommended for ease of use and accuracy)
- Ingredient list (optional, but recommended as a safety precaution and also nice to have when trying to replicate the recipe at a later date)

- External use (essential if ingredients should not be ingested)
- Contraindications (essential if formulation should not be used by people with particular medical issues, who are taking medications, or who are pregnant or nursing, etc.)

Additional.Information.to.Include.on.Labels.

Salves & Lip Balms
- Recommended application method and frequency
- Instructions for proper storage and shelf life
- Any specific precautions or warnings for sensitive skin or allergies

Teas
- Brewing instructions, including water temperature and steeping time
- Recommended serving size or number of cups per day
- Additional ingredients that can be added for flavor or benefits

Culinary Products
- May need nutritional guidelines breakdowns, with calorie and vitamins listed. It is a requirement in many places. Fortunately, there are plenty of websites provide free nutrition calculators.

Legal Considerations

- Decide on a legal structure for your business (e.g., sole proprietorship, LLC) and register it accordingly. It is easy to do it online.
- Stay updated on tax obligations, business licenses, intellectual property protection, and other legal requirements.
- Understand home business regulations.
- Check county housing regulations if housing interns.
- Get liability insurance (usually requiring a million-dollar coverage for edible products).
- Explore Farm Direct Sales guidelines, which may offer exemptions from costly requirements like commercial kitchens.
- Note that topical products do not require licensing.
- Learn the rules between independent contractors who you pay cash and employees who need payroll tax deducted.
- Keep detailed financial records and consider hiring an accountant or using accounting software.
- Get tax advice before you need it.
- If you state you are organic on labels or marketing, you need to meet the standards set by the National Organic Program (NOP) within the U.S. Department of Agriculture (USDA).
- Keep receipts of all your product purchases so you can show they are organic.
- Navigate FDA rules and state regulations meticulously.
- Talk to other herbal entrepreneurs on what legal issues they have run into, even if they make different products.

Compliance with Regulatory Bodies

In the United States, herbalists can provide herbal information and preparations for educational purposes without requiring a specific licensing mechanism. If you sell products that will be ingested, you will need to be aware of the rules regarding them. Regulations prohibit the use of marketing language that suggests herbal products *diagnose, treat, cure, or prevent diseases.* This extends to structure/function claims, which describe how nutrients or ingredients affect the human body's normal structure or function. You can use words like support, soothe, balance or ease instead of words such as cure, treat or heal.

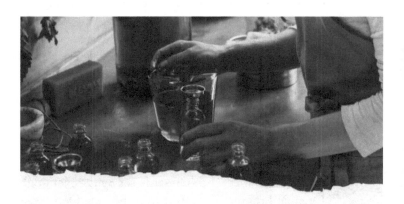

Say this: $\longrightarrow$	Instead of this:
Ease	Relieve
Soothe	Reduce
Herbal	Medicinal
Support	Heal
Balance	Treat
Aches	Pain
Occasional swelling	Inflammation
Seasonal/occasional	Chronic
Minor	Serious/intense

Photo from Herbal Content Cottage

In order to sell tinctures or similar products, you will need to meet regulations known as the Current Good Manufacturing Practices (cGMPs). Check out the American Herbalist Guild <u>website</u> for legal and regulatory FAQs.

In the early days, Eagletree Herbs was tiny, regulatory oversight was minimal, and medical claims appeared on many product labels from that era, including most of mine. Once I got a commercial kitchen license, scrutiny from the Oregon State Health Division became a significant factor. Adherence to guidelines became non-negotiable to avoid penalties or closure. I had to relabel many products and amend advertising across my website and Etsy store. I also had to stop selling many products. Dealing with all the various rules and regulations contributed to my decision to retire from the business.

While navigating these regulations can be burdensome, agencies like the FDA exist for a reason. Where they fall short is in distinguishing between products that support health (like plants) and those intended to treat disease (like drugs).

If you want to have a business that makes money, you need to work within their guidelines. It will take an initial investment of time and money to take the cGMP course and learn how to follow the rules, but you just need to be aware from the beginning and plan accordingly. Some people choose to only focus on topicals for this reason. It is sometimes possible to hire someone to come in and help you get set up, and you can go on from there.

One of the best resources is the <u>American Herbal Product Association</u> (AHPA), the professional association for those who make herbal products. Their site is chock full of valuable resource and guides you will need to follow the guidelines.

Advantages in Starting an Herbal Business

- Creates resilience systems.
- Encourages barter.
- Extra products can be donated to Community Clinics.
- May use resources otherwise wasted (like weeds).
- Supports a holistic and healthy lifestyle.
- Vending at events is a great social experience and way to connect with your community.
- Herbal medicine making skills are valuable in homesteading and survival situations.
- Being your own boss.
- Making your own hours.
- Learning new skills.
- Creating a job you are passionate about.
- Learn skills useful in other areas of business.
- Can be a healthy, fun and family activity.

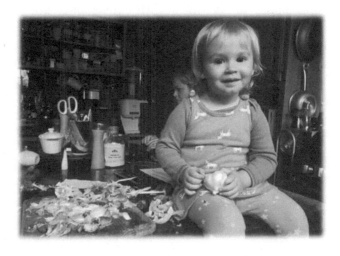

Granddaughter Coral peeling garlic for medicine

Vending is a wonderful way to market your business, connect with community, meet people, and do market research.

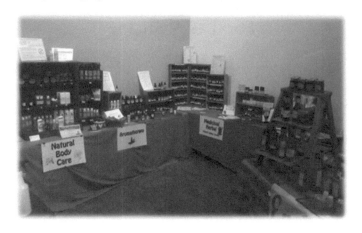

Sprout Farmers Market 2013

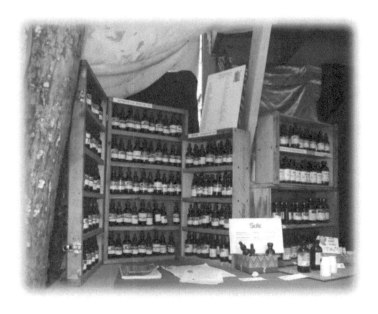

We had cases custom made that we could fold and carry. A game changer for transporting and set-up times.

Chapter Three
Food as Medicine

Learning about herbs is learning about health. It starts with food. Whole, nutritious foods contain vitamins, minerals, antioxidants, fiber, protein, and fat, essential for promoting health and optimal bodily function. Nutritional deficiencies contribute to inflammation and diseases. Diets rich in highly processed foods, laden with unhealthy additives, sugars, and fats, often lack essential nutrients because of excessive processing. In our fast-paced society, convenience often supersedes health and sustainability in food choices.

Highly processed foods often contain chemicals and other unhealthy ingredients. They also contribute to the corporate food conglomerates that contribute to the biodiversity loss and environmental degradation.

Many people explore alternative diets like vegan, keto, or paleo, each with potential health benefits, but rigid adherence can lead to stress, guilt, and added expense. Blue Zones, where people live longest and healthiest, emphasize a predominantly plant-based diet with minimal meat and dairy,

Indigenous people traditionally ate foods that grew around them, and some were more plant based than others. There are lessons to be learned there. As far as I know, there are no Indigenous people or tribes anywhere in the world that lived solely on a vegan diet. Diet discipline is a good thing, as long as it does not become like a dogmatic religion you try to convert everyone else too. Diet and food choices are very personal and should be respected. Many people, after much study, choose the Flexitarian Diet for being simple and easy.

Flexitarian Diet

1. Eat Mostly Plants:
Emphasize grains, beans,
fruits, and vegetables.

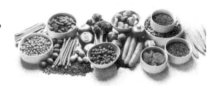

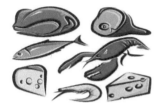

2. Occasionally Things that Eat Plants: Dairy, meat, fish, and eggs in moderation.

3. Avoid Foods Made in Plants:
such as factory-made foods,
including highly processed plant-
based meats and dairy products.

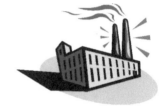

Plants Contain Phytonutrients *(or phytochemicals)*

- Produced by plants and found in various parts like roots, barks, stems, leaves, flowers, nuts, and seeds.
- Known for their health benefits, including anti-inflammatory, antioxidant, anti-aging, and anti-cancer properties.
- Whole, unprocessed or minimally processed plants are most effective, as they contain synergistic compounds that isolated phytonutrients may lack.

Foods that Boost Immune System

- Fermented Foods (e.g., kombucha, kimchi)
- Yogurt and Kefir
- Garlic and Onions
- Nettles
- Citrus Fruits, Bell Peppers
- Cruciferous Vegetables (e.g., broccoli, spinach, kale)
- Bone Broth
- Ginger and Turmeric
- Berries (e.g., blueberries, elderberries)
- Fire Cider

Is Eating Healthy Only for the Privileged?

- Expense of restricted diets (e.g., organic, vegan, gluten-free) unless homegrown or limited.
- Time-consuming nature of preparing healthy meals, especially for working individuals.
- Inequities in food access for lower-income communities living in food deserts.
- Socioeconomic factors can influence generational dietary habits.

Childhood Trauma & Food

Adverse childhood experiences (ACEs) correlate with high-risk health behaviors, such as smoking, drug use, and obesity. Food insecurity during childhood impacts lifelong relationships with food, often leading to emotional eating and unhealthy coping mechanisms. Awareness of trauma-related behaviors is crucial for fostering a healthy relationship with food. There also can be generational unhealthy eating patterns. While you may not have ever experienced hunger as a child, if a parent or even a grandparent did, it may affect you.

Food Addiction

- Addiction to specific diets can mimic unhealthy behaviors if they become obsessive.
- Certain foods, particularly fats, activate brain pleasure centers similar to drugs.
- Overeating may disrupt satiety signals in the brain, contributing to weight gain and related health issues.

Growing Food Combats Inequities

- Gardening promotes food sovereignty, empowering individuals to reclaim control over their food sources.
- Enhances community engagement and resilience against corporate food systems reliant on industrial practices and fossil fuels.

Gardening Improves Health

- Provides gentle exercise, enhancing strength, balance, and promoting better sleep.
- Exposure to sunlight boosts vitamin D production, critical for immune function.
- Horticulture therapy shows cognitive benefits and mood enhancement because of soil microorganisms with antidepressant qualities.

Eating seasonally supports local agriculture and ensures fresher, more nutritious food choices. For example:

- **Spring**: Asparagus, strawberries, and leafy greens.
- **Summer**: Tomatoes, cucumbers, and berries.
- **Fall**: Squash, apples, and root vegetables.
- **Winter**: Citrus fruits, Brussels sprouts, and kale.

Ancestral, Cultural, and Ethnic Perspectives

Some evidence suggests ethnic-specific diets may better suit genetic predispositions and metabolic needs. Different cultural diets offer unique health benefits and preserve culinary traditions.

Examples include:

- **Mediterranean Diet**: Rich in fruits, vegetables, whole grains, and healthy fats like olive oil, it has been linked to reduced risk of heart disease.
- **Traditional Japanese Diet**: High in fish, rice, vegetables, and fermented foods, it promotes longevity.
- **Latin American Diet**: Incorporates beans, corn, and a variety of fresh produce, providing a balanced nutritional profile.
- **Diets rich in Spices and Herbs**: like Indian cuisine, are known for its use of turmeric and ginger for their anti-inflammatory properties.
- **Indigenous Traditional Food Diets:** depending on the tribe may have a diet heavy in meat, wild rice, salmon or other fish, corn and beans, whale or other wild caught foods.

Traditional Chinese Medicine (TCM) and Ayurveda:

- Foods are categorized by their energetic properties, such as "cold", "damp", or "hot". For example, beets are considered cool and sweet, which can help calm the heart.
- Adapting the diet to the seasons, such as nourishing the liver in spring and the lungs in fall.
- Emphasizing freshness, lightly cooking vegetables, and pre-soaking beans and grains.
- Eating larger meals earlier in the day.
- Drinking warm water or herbal tea before meals and eating warm, cooked foods to support digestion.

Mindful Eating Practices

Practicing mindful eating involves paying full attention to the experience of eating and drinking.

Benefits include:

- **Improved Digestion**: Eating slowly and chewing thoroughly aids digestion.
- **Better Food Appreciation**: Noticing flavors and textures can enhance enjoyment.
- **Awareness of Hunger Cues**: Being mindful helps distinguish between physical hunger and emotional eating.
- **Pray or Express Gratitude**: For the growers and preparers of food.
- **Do Not Eat in Front of the TV or Phone**: I am guilty of that, probably is one reason I am fat.
- **Have Family Dinners:** Research shows children who sit with their parent/s for at least one meal a day do better in school and other measurements of well-being.

Dietary needs vary with age and life stages

1. **Infants:** Need breastmilk for the first year, if unavailable infant formula.
2. **Children**: Require nutrients for growth and development, such as calcium and protein.
3. **Adults**: Need balanced diets to maintain health and prevent chronic diseases.
4. **Pregnant and Lactating Women**: Need additional calories, vitamins, minerals, and foods rich in iron and calcium.
5. **Elders**: Benefit from foods rich in calcium, vitamin D, and fiber to support bone health and digestion.

Environmental Impact of Food Choices

- While reducing meat consumption can lower greenhouse gas emissions in factory farm meat, grazing animals can have benefits to the environment when done responsibly.
- Monoculture farming practices cause biodiversity loss.
- Eating locally grown foods in season supports regional farming and reduces transportation emissions.
- Growing and preserving your own food through canning, freezing, or fermenting can be healthy and cost efficient, and help reduce your carbon footprint.
- Eating and supporting organic foods reduces pesticides that enter the entire ecosystem and kill bees. Bees are vital to the survival of the planet and humans and are crucial for biodiversity and health. They are pollinators that move pollen between the male and female parts of flowers, which is the first step in creating seeds and new plants.

Community Food Initiatives

Supporting local food systems strengthens communities and ensures food security. **Examples include**:

- **Community Gardens**: Neighborhood gardens where residents can grow their own food.
- **Farmer's Markets**: Local markets that provide fresh, seasonal produce.
- **Food Cooperatives**: Member-owned businesses that sell groceries and emphasize local and sustainable products.
- **Gleaning Groups**: Harvesting and preserving food that might normally be thrown out.

Food Justice and Advocacy

Efforts to address food insecurity and promote equitable access to nutritious food include:

- **Food Banks and Pantries**: Providing free groceries to those in need.
- **School Lunch Programs**: Ensuring children receive nutritious meals at school.
- **Advocacy Organizations**: Groups like Feeding America work to combat hunger and improve food policies.

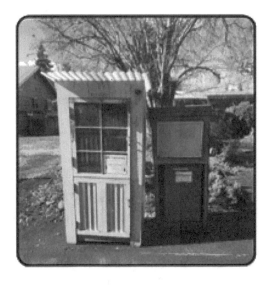

Little Library, Food Pantry and Free Fridge in front of Daphne's house in Eugene, Oregon.

Easy way to share food and get to know your neighbors.

What Is Food Sovereignty?

Food sovereignty is a food system in which the people who produce, distribute, and consume food also control the mechanisms and policies of food production and distribution. This stands in contrast to the present corporate food regime, in which corporations and market institutions control the global food system.

It also is the right and ability of **tribal** nations and peoples to cultivate, access, and secure nutritious, **culturally essential food** produced through ecologically sound and sustainable methods.

Indigenous tribes are moving toward this goal though restoring fishing and hunting rights, growing and gathering food.

All people can move towards food sovereignty by becoming less dependent on corporate food systems which rely on factories and fossil fuels.

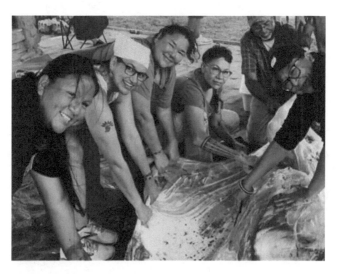

Linda Black Elk, Indigenous ethnobotanist and food sovereignty activist with the Standing Rock tribe at traditional buffalo harvest.

Chapter Four
Transforming Plants to Medicines

Two Methods of Making Herbal Medicines

1. Folk Method

Based on tradition and handed down through generations, individuals can learn the folk method from their family or through apprenticeship. Indigenous people of the Americas have an extensive wisdom of plant medicine, which forms the basis of much of our herbal knowledge today. In South America, there is significant research now on finding plants that may cure serious 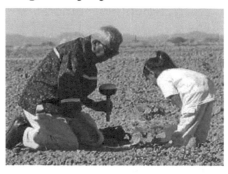 diseases. Unfortunately, in North America, the cultural genocide that occurred with the boarding school generation led to much information being lost or not passed down. Many Native people today must reacquire herbal knowledge from other sources. In addition to knowledge by Indigenous peoples, there is a rich body of knowledge held by Celtic and European peoples over the centuries, often referred to as Wise Woman teachings. Herbalists and midwives, who may have been persecuted as witches, primarily utilized this knowledge of healing with plants, which was seen as a threat to male authority powers. African, Asian, and Middle Eastern cultures have a rich trove of plant medicine traditions.

The folk method includes qualities not always understood by science or based on understood facts. There may be spiritual or magical properties in plants or methods of harvesting or preparation. For example, people may harvest some herbs in certain cycles of the moon. In some traditions, a woman on her menstrual cycle would not prepare medicines intended for a man. There may be prayers, rituals, or gifts given to plants being harvested.

The benefit of this method is that each product is unique and may contain the power of the intention, love, and attention of the medicine maker. This method may not use exact recipes, relying instead on rough quantities and using smell, taste, and texture to create.

2. Scientific Method

The scientific method uses exact recipes with consistent quantities of each ingredient, harvested in the same way each time. This method proves ideal for products that will be sold. It has the advantage of the ability to measure and reproduce results exactly each time. This method is especially useful for research and evidence-based medicine.

To conduct research and evidence-based medicine, one needs science. If we are to find out which herbs are good for what conditions, we need a consistent basis for comparison.

Herbal pharmacognosy is the application of this science specifically to traditional herbal medicine sources. This method studies complex compounds such as phytochemicals that create mechanisms of action that modulate physiological functions.

- Use exact written recipes.
- Use consistent quantities of each ingredient.
- Harvested the same way each time.
- If buying herbs, use the same source if possible.
- Label accurately.

Guidelines on the Use of Medicinal Plants

Proper Identification: Many plants bear a resemblance to each other. It is crucial to confirm the identity of plants using at least two sources: a knowledgeable person and an objective reference like a book, a photograph from the internet, or a plant identification app on your phone. Numerous plant apps are available for phones, offering ease and speed in identification. Some poisonous plants closely resemble medicinal ones, underscoring the importance of absolute certainty. It is advisable to own a couple of reliable plant identification books and seek confirmation from multiple sources if there is any doubt.

Local Names and Varieties: Local names can be ambiguous, as several plants may share the same name. For instance, "Yerba Buena," which translates to "good herb," is used for several different plants. Similarly, herbs with similar names, such as "heal all" and "self-heal," may refer to different botanical species.

Understanding Plant Parts and Usage: It is essential to know which part of the plant to use whether it is the leaf, root, flower, or sometimes, the whole plant—since each part may possess different medicinal properties. It is crucial to check if there are specific guidelines for their use, such as using only fresh parts.

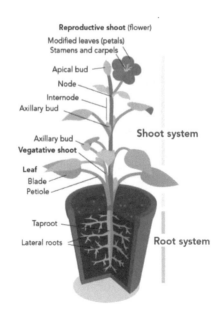

Reproductive shoot (flower)
Modified leaves (petals)
Stamens and carpels
Apical bud
Node
Internode
Axillary bud
Axillary bud
Vegatative shoot
Leaf
Blade
Petiole
Taproot
Lateral roots
Shoot system
Root system

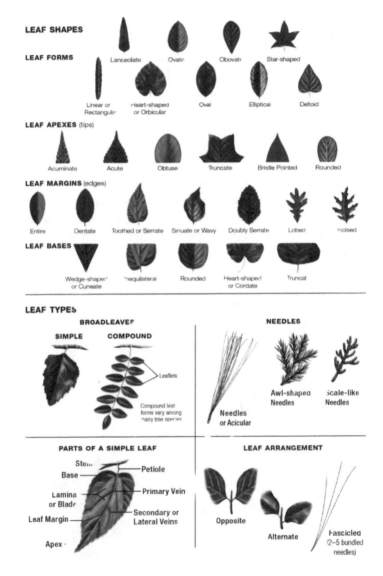

LEAF SHAPES

LEAF FORMS

Lanceolate   Ovate   Obovate   Star-shaped

Linear or Rectangular   Heart-shaped or Orbicular   Oval   Elliptical   Deltoid

LEAF APEXES (tips)

Acuminate   Acute   Obtuse   Truncate   Bristle Pointed   Rounded

LEAF MARGINS (edges)

Entire   Dentate   Toothed or Serrate   Sinuate or Wavy   Doubly Serrate   Lobed   Incised

LEAF BASES

Wedge-shaped or Cuneate   Inequilateral   Rounded   Heart-shaped or Cordate   Truncate

LEAF TYPES

BROADLEAVES

SIMPLE   COMPOUND

Leaflets

Compound leaf forms vary among many tree species

NEEDLES

Awl-shaped Needles   Scale-like Needles

Needles or Acicular

PARTS OF A SIMPLE LEAF

Stem   Petiole
Base
Lamina or Blade   Primary Vein
Leaf Margin   Secondary or Lateral Veins
Apex

LEAF ARRANGEMENT

Opposite

Alternate

Fascicled (2–5 bundled needles)

Preparations to Make Medicines

Maintain Cleanliness: Maintain strict cleanliness standards when handling medicinal plant materials. Clean and sanitize all surfaces, utensils, and tools using bleach or other sanitizing solutions, following the practices used in commercial kitchens.

Create a Medicine Making Space: Ideally have a dedicated space, but if you use your own kitchen, remove all personal food, and clean thoroughly. Be aware of nut allergies. Even the slightest bit of something like peanut butter left on your counter could cause a reaction.

Choose Suitable Cooking Utensils: Avoid using aluminum, iron, tin, or other metals, as they can leach into your products.

Use Pure Water: Use filtered or distilled water.

Prepare Jars and Lids in Advance: Make sure you clean, check for proper fit, and prepare all jars and lids before starting. This prevents last-minute issues during the pouring process.

Ensure Proper Identification, Harvesting, Preparation, and Labeling: Thoroughly identify, harvest, prepare, and label all materials, particularly for medicinal products.

Document Your Recipes: Maintain written records of your recipes to ensure consistency in product replication. This practice prevents forgetting exact measurements between production runs. In writing this book, I could only include the recipes that were written down. There were many products I made decades ago left out.

Pray or Create Intentions: Positive energy and affirmation can help imbue the spirit of the plants into your medicines and products.

Harvesting Herbs

Right Time of Year to Collect

- **Leaves**—Gather when the plant is about to bloom.
- **Flowers**—Harvest just before or shortly after they open.
- **Seeds**—Collect after the fruits have fully matured.
- **Roots**—Best harvested in early spring or late fall.
- **Barks**—Gather before sap rises, in very early spring or late fall.

Right Time of Day to Collect

- Ideally, in the morning after the dew has evaporated.
- Before the hot sun dissipates essential oils, typically between 10 am and 12 pm on a dry day.

Right Place to Collect

- Ensure the area is free from pesticides or chemicals.
- Avoid locations near busy roadways and car exhaust.
- Harvest where plants are plentiful and not endangered or over-harvested. Always leave enough for next year's harvest.

Four steps in traditional method of harvesting plants
(how I was taught, many traditions exist)

- ❖ **Step One**—Ask for Permission.
- ❖ **Step Two**—Bring an Offering.
- ❖ **Step Three**—Take only what you need, leave enough for the plant & others.
- ❖ **Step Four**—Give thanks, gratitude for the life spirit in plants.

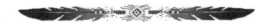

Post-Harvest Preparation

"Garbling" or breaking down into smaller or more usable forms.

- Prepare herbs by discarding brown, decayed, or poor-quality parts.
- Separate and remove unwanted materials such as stems and midribs from leaves, or dirt and foreign matter.

Roots

- Scrub thoroughly with a brush and warm water until clean.
- Roots are easier to chop when fresh before drying.

Washing Leaves & Flowers

- Wash if there's a risk of contamination (e.g., from dog urine) or bugs, though not always necessary.
- Quickly rinse with cool water to avoid washing away essential oils.
- Excess water can lead to mold during drying, depending on the method used.

Drying Herbs

Air Drying

- Choose a well-shaded, well-ventilated area.

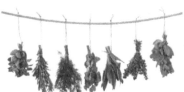

- Methods include screens, baskets, or hanging bunches with rubber bands that shrink as they dry.

Dehydrators

- Home kitchen units.
- Commercial models.
- Solar (as long as herbs are shaded)
- Dry at less than 140 degrees unless thick leaves like mullein.

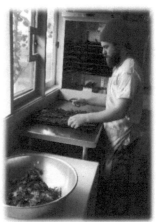

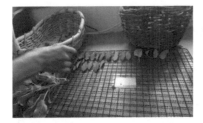

After Drying

Milling—reduction to the required particle size can be done by hand or with tools.

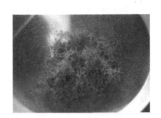

Sieving—to collect the required uniformly sized particles.

Straining—to remove big stems or other unwanted parts.

Grinding—hand grinders, coffee grinders, mortar and pestle.

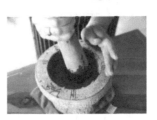

Break down enough to not allow too much air into storage containers but do not powder or break down too much prior to use.

Storage

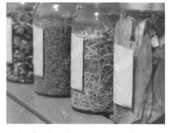

- Glass over plastic; use dark or colored glass if only clear glass is available or cover clear glass with paper.
- Seal tightly and store in a cool, dark place away from sunlight.
- Use desiccants or charcoal inside containers to absorb moisture for thick herbs.
- Properly label containers with the plant name, collection date, and location.

For Medicinal Use, Label with:

- Conditions treated.
- Preparation method.
- Usage instructions or dosage.
- Contraindications or special precautions.
- Storage and expiry dates.

For medicines you should label:

- Conditions it is used for
- Method of preparation
- Directions for use or dosage
- Contraindication/Special Precautions
- Storage Date
- Expiration Date

Properly dried and stored plants maintain quality for one season or one year.

Chapter Five
Making Products

Why Make Your Own Herbal Products?

Quality—The best way to ensure the highest quality possible is to make it yourself. If having all organically grown ingredients is important to you, only select those ingredients. While you may need to make occasional compromises to balance costs, you control those decisions.

Freshness—Ideally, you can grow or wild harvest the herbs to ensure maximum freshness. Even if you must buy herbs from an herbal vendor, you can look at the dates and know how old the herbs are that go into your products. When you buy a pre-made product, you do not know how old the herbs or other ingredients are.

Cost-Effective—It costs pennies on the dollar to make your own products. For example, a typical two-ounce bottle of lemon balm tincture is $18. If you grow your own lemon balm, which is easy to grow, the cost is just your time to harvest it. If you must buy it, two ounces of lemon balm costs about $5. A quart of alcohol, depending on whether you use low-cost vodka or organic alcohol, will run between $10 and $20. For the cost of one two-ounce bottle, you can make an entire quart.

Easy—If you can cook, you can make herbal products. There are lots of recipes online besides this book, and while there may be an occasional product that is more difficult, it is usually straightforward.

Fun—Turning plants into medicines and other products involves hands-on learning and creativity. There is joy in hand making medicines and gifts. Doing it with friends and family can make it even more enjoyable.

Infusions

Infusions are Hot Teas

While you may serve it chilled, it's recommended to take infusions prepared for colds and flu hot. Infusions are used for leaves, flowers, and tender herbs.

Making Infusions

1. Pour 1 cup of boiling water over 1 tablespoon of dry herb, or 1 ounce of dried herb for every pint of hot water.
2. If fresh herbs are used, use three times the amount of dried.
3. Cover with a lid and allow herbs to steep for 15-20 minutes. Leaving the lid off will let important essential oils escape.
4. Strain and drink. Can be stored in the refrigerator for 1-2 days.

Standard dosage: One cup three times a day. Can be made stronger for a more medicinal effect.

Nourishing infusions: ½ cup nourishing herb such as nettles or milky oat, a quart of boiling water and allowed to sit overnight and drank cold the next day.

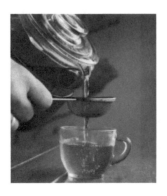

Decoctions

Decoctions are boiled teas

Best method for barks, seeds, nuts, and roots.

Decoctions extract primarily mineral salts and bitter principles rather than vitamins and volatile ingredients.

Making Decoctions

1. Boil 1 cup of water (ideally in a nonmetal pot) with 1tablespoon of dry herb, or 1 ounce of dried herb for every pint of hot water. If you use a fresh plant, use three times the amount of dried herb. Break up large pieces of materials into smaller pieces.
2. Cover and simmer on low for 25-45 minutes. After simmering will be about ¾ the amount of water volume.
3. Strain and drink.

Can be stored in the refrigerator for 1-2 days.

Standard Dosage: One cup three times a day. Can be made stronger for a more medicinal effect. If the herb is very bitter or strong, use 4 teaspoons three times a day.

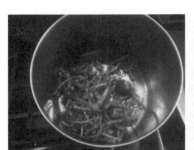
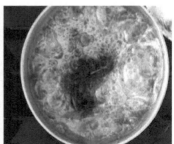

Cold Extract

Preparing herbs with cold water preserves the most volatile ingredients while extracting only minor amounts of mineral salts and bitter principles. Used often for mucilaginous herbs that form a gel-like consistency when mixed with water. It is

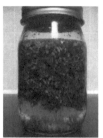

common for people to use it with mucilaginous herbs like marshmallow root and slippery elm, which are wonderful for soothing the throat, digestive tract, and urinary tract irritation. People traditionally use them externally as a poultice for minor burns and wounds.

Method of Preparation: Maceration
1. Measure 2 tablespoons of dried or 6 tablespoons of fresh plants in one cup of water.
2. Put the herbs in a glass or ceramic container.
3. Macerate for about 8 to 12 hours.
4. Strain and put in a storage glass bottle.
5. Store in the refrigerator for 1-2 days.

Standard Dosage: One cup three times a day. Can be strengthened for a more medicinal effect.

Ultrasonic Extraction

Ultra sonication is an extraction technique using ultrasound waves from a machine. Sonication breaks the cell structure and releases the bioactive compounds—resulting in higher yields and faster extraction rates. It is supposed to yield undamaged bioactive compounds, preserving valuable phytochemicals. Instead of using the expensive machines designed for this, an herbalist friend of mine used an ultrasonic jewelry cleaning machine. The end product does not keep well. It would be harder to market, but in some situations, may have value.

Tinctures or Extracts

The term "tincture" refers to concentrated herbal extracts. People often use the terms tincture/extract interchangeably, but technically, only a tincture uses alcohol as the solvent. If you are using vinegar, glycerin, or any menstruum (solvent) other than alcohol, your preparation is an extract.

To make them, you place fresh or dried herbs into a jar and cover them with a solvent (menstruum): alcohol, glycerin, or vinegar. After sealing the mixture, let it macerate (soak) for 2-6 weeks.

Tinctures or extracts can increase the bioavailability of specific herbal constituents, which are hard to access in the dried or raw form. They also offer concentration, ease of use, and convenience, lasting many years.

Alcohol is the most common menstruum.
- It dissolves the most active constituents out of the plant matter.
- Acts as a preservative, keeping its effectiveness for years.
- It is possible to use any part of the plant, whether it is dried or fresh.
- Can be made with vodka, 180 proof "Everclear" or 100% cane or grain alcohol.
- Dilute 100% alcohol by 50% with distilled water.

How to Make an Alcohol Tincture

Different people use different ratios. A 1 in 5 ratio for dried herbs is most often used in commercially sold tinctures and recommended by some medicine makers. I recommend using a 1-4 ratio, preferring a slightly stronger tincture.

Using **dried herbs**, use 1-part dried herb (broke down finely but not powdered), to 4-parts alcohol for a 1:4 ratio. When you add alcohol, dried herbs will expand, so make sure to leave room in the jar.

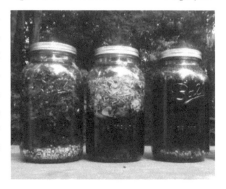

For **fresh herbs**, use equal parts herbs to alcohol.1:2 ratio.

1. Place in a glass jar, alcohol should freely cover herbs. Herbs not covered with alcohol could mold or spoil.
2. Cover tightly. A canning jar lid works well, but if left over six weeks may affect metal lids, so some people use a piece of parchment paper under the lid.
3. Store in a cool dark place and shake daily.
4. After four to six weeks, strain (French press works great), discard plant matter, label, and use the tincture.
5. Store at room temperature away from direct sunlight.

Tips for matching your alcohol strength to the herb being tinctured *(from Mountain Rose Herbs)*

40% to 50% alcohol by volume (80- to 90-proof vodka) "Standard" percentage range for tinctures.

Good for:
- Most dried herbs and fresh herbs that are not super juicy.
- And extraction of water-soluble properties.

67.5% to 70% alcohol by volume (half 80-proof vodka and half 190-proof grain alcohol). Extracts the most volatile aromatic properties.

Good for:

- Fresh, high-moisture herbs like lemon balm, berries, and aromatic roots. The higher alcohol percentage will draw out more of the plant juices.

85% to 95% alcohol by volume (190-proof grain alcohol). This alcohol strength can produce a tincture that's difficult to take and will also dehydrate the herbs if used for botanicals beyond gums and resins.

Good for:

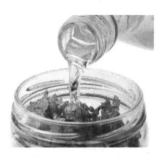

- Dissolving gums and resins but unnecessary for most plant material.
- Extracts the aromatics and essential oils bound in a plant that doesn't dissipate easily.

Making Tincture Blends

Combining several tinctures to treat specific conditions, such as for sleep, or urinary tract infections, can be highly effective as well as convenient. Also called formulations.

While some herbalists tincture all herbs designed for a blend in one jar, I prefer to make each one individually and then mix them. This has the advantage of being able to taste and try each individual herb for strength and quality.

Creating your own formulations is an art and a science. While evidence-based is good practice, sometimes intuition and instinct are part of the process.

Some people use herbs that grow together, while others use Eastern philosophy of herbs that are "cold" or "warm" or that apply to specific individual constitutions.

Do not use the "kitchen sink" method of making blends, that is, throw everything but the kitchen sink in. I use four to seven of most herbs and try to find ones that will balance and complement each other. The Eagletree blends are in the recipe section. You are free to use these or develop your own, experiment, and find the best ones for you.

Glycerites

Vegetable glycerin is a clear, odorless, sweet-tasting, fatty liquid that comes from vegetable fats and oils, such as coconut, soybean, or palm. It's also known as glycerol or glyceryl triacetate. Glycerin is a useful menstruum for children or those who cannot have alcohol, or people in recovery. Glycerin can extract for some oil soluble constituents that do not extract with alcohol (cannabis).

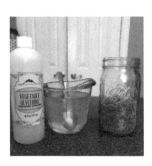

How to Make a Glycerin Tincture

1. Fill a mason jar ½ way with dried herbs. Using dried herbs (broken down finely but not powdered), double the amount of fresh herbs.
2. In a separate jar, mix 3 parts vegetable glycerin and 1 part distilled water. Shake to combine (some sources use different ratios).
3. Pour liquid mixture over the herb and completely cover to fill the jar.
4. Label container with date, ratio of glycerin to water, and herbs used.
5. Shake daily for 4-6 weeks.
6. Strain, discard plant matter, label, and use.
7. Refrigerate or store in a cool place away from direct sunlight.

Glycerites keep for 6 months to a year.

Quick Method for Glycerin Tinctures

Using this method may lose some alkaloids sensitive to heat, however by taste and smell this method is stronger.

1. Place in a glass jar, put the jar in a crock pot with a washcloth in the pot's bottom to keep it from scorching.
2. Fill the crock pot with water, making a double boiler with the jar of glycerin and herbs.
3. Cover tightly and put on the lowest setting for three days, adding water in the crock pot as needed. Turn or shake periodically.
4. After three days, strain, discard plant matter, label, and use.

Percolation Tincture

Percolation tinctures are common in traditional Chinese medicine. The method uses alcohol to dehydrate and break down the plant's cell wall, allowing the preserving menstruum to extract the medicinal properties of the plant. It uses powdered or finely ground herbs.

1. Moisten herbs with your menstruum (alcohol/water).
2. Let it sit for 12-24 hours to moisten and expand.
3. Pack it into a cone (not too gently, or too hard)
4. Pour the remainder of the menstruum over the herb, allowing it to slowly drip out.
5. Water extracts only last a few days, alcohol will last years.

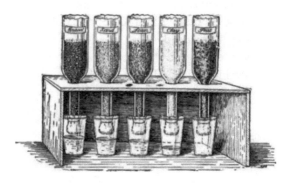

Herbal Vinegars

Can be used as food or
medicine. Great for
tonics (herbs to take daily
to build the immune
system and keep healthy).
Apple Cider Vinegar is
best if you use one with
the "mother" which is
loaded with probiotics.

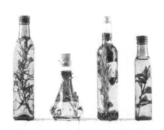

1. Using dried herbs, use 1-part dried herb (broken down finely but not powdered), to 3 parts vinegar. Double the amount of fresh herbs.
2. Place in a glass jar, put the jar in a warm place such as a sunny window, but place the jar in a paper bag or cover it, to keep it dark.
3. Cover tightly and turn or shake periodically.
4. After two weeks strain with cheesecloth, discard plant matter and label and use, or keep plants in.

Fire Cider

Is a traditional herbal vinegar, used extensively to boost the immune system and treat several respiratory conditions. Typically made with herbs like garlic, onions, ginger, turmeric, citrus, thyme, horseradish, and usually hot peppers like cayenne. Recipes vary and it is good to make to your own taste. Most often made with honey, adding the benefits of honey and helps the taste. Since honey, being antiseptic, can kill some probiotics, some make it without it. We made a traditional fire cider called Dragon's Breath recipe on page 116. We also made a variation of fire cider called Tonigrette, with nettles that is fantastic for the immune system. It does not have honey to boost the probiotics.

Oxymels

Made by infusing in vinegar and honey—used most often with pungent or strong herbs. Fire Cider is an oxymel, although some say oxymels are only those with equal parts honey.

- 1 part vinegar
- 1 part honey
- Dried herbs (like thyme, garlic, oregano, sage, ginger, and cayenne)

You can make infused vinegar, and infused honey separately and mix the two after you have infused them, or you can make at the same time and save a step. The advantage of making one at a time is to make a stand-alone product. For example, you can make hot honey with cayenne, add it to another herbal vinegar and use just hot honey by itself (it is great on toast).

1. Fill a jar ¼ full of dried herbs, then fill the rest of the jar with equal parts honey and vinegar.
2. Stir the mixture, then place a lid on the jar and shake well.
3. Place the jar in a cool, dark area and allow it to infuse for two to four weeks.
4. Shake it periodically.
5. After soaking time is complete, strain the herbs, pour into a jar, and label it.

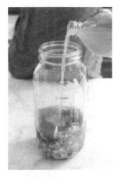 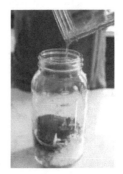

Honey & Electuaries

Infuse **herbal honey** in the same way you make herbal oils, either by covering it in the sun or using a crock-pot. They are strained and then used.

Electuaries are herbs mixed with honey or other sweeteners. The herbs are eaten as a paste without straining. Honey has a lot of powerful healing properties on its own, and herbs add to its usefulness.

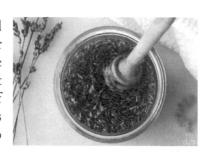

Syrups and Elixirs

Herbal syrups are concentrated solutions of sugar & herbs in aqueous fluids. Elixirs are syrups with alcohol. Ideal for herbs used as medicine with an unpleasant taste. Elixirs are 50% syrup or honey and 25-50% tincture. Syrups soothe and are good for cough and throat mixtures. Standard dosage is one teaspoon three times a day.

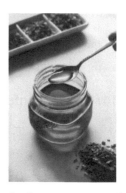

Cane sugar is a good preservative and does not need additional preservation. Honey can also serve as a preservative. However, if you add water to honey, it will ferment, and you must refrigerate it. Alcohol serves as an additional preservative option. Syrups need to be preserved with 20% alcohol or canned using the water bath method.

How to Make Herbal Syrup (makes 1000 mL of Syrup)

1. Use only granulated sugar in the correct quantity, if in too small a proportion, fermentation is apt to occur. If too abundant, crystallization.
2. Make your herbal decoction or infusion and strain well.
3. Measure 465 ml of fluid. While the mixture is hot, add 850g of sugar and let it boil until you achieve the desired consistency.
4. Pour into a clean glass jar while hot, bottle and seal.
5. Allow to cool prior to use.

Infused Oils

Oils infused with herbs are good for topical application (external use). Also used as an ingredient for salves, ointments, lotions or creams. Can be prepared by hot or cold methods. Choose an oil with good storage results, such as olive oil or coconut oil. Use only very dry herbs, moisture in the oil might cause mold to grow.

How to Make Infused Oil Method 1 (Hot Method)

1. Place in a glass or enameled-coated container 1 cup dried herbs and cover with 2 cups oil.
2. Place jar in a crock pot with a washcloth in the bottom of the pot to keep it from scorching.
3. Fill the crock pot with water, essentially making a double boiler with the jar of oil and herbs.
4. Cover jar tightly and put on the lowest setting for 24 hours, adding water to the crock pot as needed. Turn or shake periodically.
5. After 24 hours, strain, and discard plant material.
6. Add 800 IU vitamin E per cup of oil as a preservative to keep the oil from becoming rancid.
7. Label properly, indicating the date of the preparation.
8. Keep it away from heat and light.

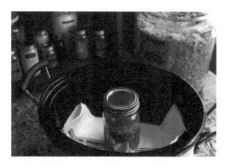

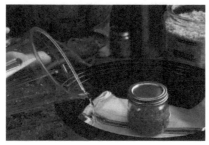

How to Make Infused Oil Method 2 (Cold Method)

Use methods described above, except instead of a crock pot, put a jar of herbs and oil in a paper bag in a sunny window for two weeks.

Ointments & Salves

Ointments and Salves do not penetrate the skin like lotions or creams but cover and protect it. They are used externally only.

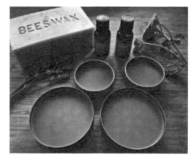

How to Make an Ointment or Salve

1. Heat 1 cup of herbal infused oil and 1 oz of beeswax in a glass or enamel-coated pan over low heat until fully melted. Stir often.
2. Once melted, remove from heat. If you are adding essential oils, add now, or if you are adding more Vitamin E or Rosemary Antioxidant as a preservative.
3. Pour the mixture into wide-mouthed glass or plastic jars before it begins to set up.
4. Allow it to cool and harden uncovered, then seal it and label it.

Liniments

Liniments help ease sore muscles, stiffness, sprains, strains, and bruising. They are used externally only.

How to Make a Liniment

1. Use 1 part infused herbal oil (for example arnica, comfrey, St John's wort) that has been previously prepared and strained.
2. 2 parts infused witch hazel or herbal tincture made with alcohol. You can also infuse herbs into rubbing alcohol.
3. Bottle and label.

Lotions & Creams

Lotion and creams are a blend of oil, beeswax and water, plus whatever herbs or essential oils you use. They absorb in the skin. Because of the water, they can harbor bacteria, and need additional care in making and additional preservatives.

Antioxidants keep oils and butters from going rancid quickly. Some examples include vitamin E and rosemary antioxidant—help slow down oxidation, so your oils won't age or smell like old oil sooner than they should but won't kill the bacteria and mold that spoils water-based products such as lotions and creams. Rosemary antioxidant is derived from the carbon dioxide extraction of rosemary leaves. It is not something you can easily make yourself and it is expensive, but very necessary.

Preservatives will kill microbes and prevent water-containing products from developing bacteria and mold quickly. Natural preservatives recommended include *Leucidal, Arborcide OC,* or *NeoDefend.* You can use good quality grapefruit seed oil, but you need to supplement it with another preservative.

After spending the time and expense of making your beautiful lotion or cream, you don't want to open it up in a month or two and find it has mold.

If a lotion or cream includes water, aloe, or any other water-based ingredient, it requires a preservative, or you should refrigerate it and use it within a few days.

How to Make a Lotion or Cream

1. Sterilize everything, jars, blender, pots. If you cannot boil, you can use a bleach solution to sterilize. Just be sure no residue remains on the equipment.
2. Use herbs prepared as glycerin tinctures, as they will add moisturizing benefits. You can also add previously made herbal infused oils.
3. Melt beeswax & oils on top of a double boiler over simmering water. Watch that the mixture gets only warm enough to melt the contents. Ensure that you blend all the ingredients well and then remove the mixture.
4. In a blender, add the water, glycerin & preservatives; add a few drops of essential oil (if desired).
5. While the blender is operating, slowly drizzle the warm melted oils and wax into the water. The mixture will become thick.
6. Pour into sterilized containers.

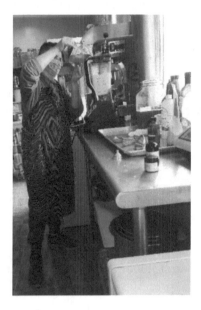
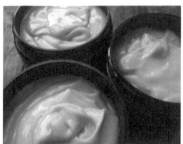

Lotion Bars

Because lotion bars contain no water, there is no need for additional preservatives.

1. Melt equal parts coconut oil, butters (cocoa or shea) and beeswax.
2. 1 teaspoon vitamin E.
3. 15-30 drops of essential oils (optional).
4. Pour into molds, then cool.

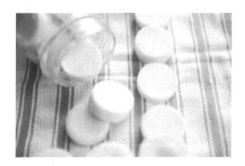

Compresses

Soak cloths in herbs and apply them externally as compresses. Or herbs in a cloth bag, then soaked in hot water then applied, like a big tea bag. When just the tea is used it is sometimes called a fomentation. Used for body aches and pains, headaches, sore throat and skin conditions. You can add tinctures of other herbs and essential oils to the liquid.

- Soak a cloth in a hot decoction/infusion of herbs, squeeze out excess liquid apply the hot cloth to the affected area.

Or

1. Make a loose bag of clean cloth the desired herb by tying with the corners or with a string.
2. Place in a bowl or pan, cover with boiling water, steep for 15–30 minutes, then let cool and apply to affected area.

Poultices

Poultices are chopped herbs applied directly to skin or through a cloth. Used for boils, abscesses, chest infections and sprains.

- Mix or chop fresh herbs in a blender or food processor. If using dried herbs pour just enough boiling water over to make a pulp.
- For hot poultices, place the pulp in a piece of cloth and apply to the affected area while hot (not burning), replace when cool.

For fresh poultices, such as comfrey for a sprain, cover the entire area with macerated plant and leave on for about an hour.

Bath Salts or Bath Bombs

Baths salts are made with Epsom or other exotic salts, some have baking soda, herbs, essential oils, or clays. Bath bombs are fun, with extra fizz. Used to soothe aches and pains, for relaxation, skin exfoliation, and mood enhancement.

Bath Bomb Basic Recipe

Ingredients:
- 1 cup baking soda
- ½ cup citric acid
- ½ cup cornstarch
- ¼ cup Epsom salt
- ¼ cup coconut oil (melted)
- 15-20 drops essential oils

You will also need a spray bottle with a little water, and bath bomb molds.

Instructions:
1. Mix the dry ingredients. Stir well.
2. Add in the melted coconut oil, essential oils, and mix.
3. Spray the mixture with water until the ingredients hold together when squeezed in your hands.
4. Press the mixture into both sides of the bath bomb molds and then put the two halves together. Wipe the excess mixture off the sides and set it aside.
5. Allow the molds to sit for 24-48 hours or until completely dry and then pop out of the molds.

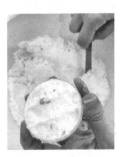
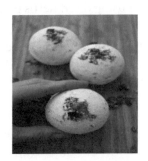

Essential Oil Misters

Essential Oils are like drugs—highly concentrated, purified, and extracted from plants. It takes about seven pounds of lavender flowers to make one ounce of essential oil.

Aromatherapy can affect the limbic system of the brain, good for anxiety, depression, and mental states. However, it is important to never take essential oils internally, as they can be toxic and even fatal if taken in large doses.

You should always use a carrier oil or dilute with distilled water. Fractionated coconut oil is a nice oil to use with essential oils as it does not go rancid like other oils and is light, with little odor by itself.

Misters

- Mix 20-40 drops for every four ounces of distilled water.
- Can use a little more if using for diffusers.
- A small amount of vodka or ethanol can be used if being used for antimicrobial.
- Use glass, as essential oils can degrade plastic. You can make misters with one essential or blend ones to have a synergetic effect.

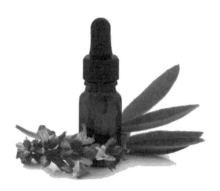

Smoking Blends

Oddly enough, smoking herbs can aid the lungs in some circumstances. Others wish to mix tobacco with herbs to reduce the nicotine and impact on the lungs.

Basic formula for smoking blends.
- 2-part base—such as mullein, raspberry leaf, or coltsfoot.
- 1 part modifier—herb that has a specific effect such for relaxation like catnip or skullcap.
- ½ part flavoring—such as mint, rose or lavender.

Steam Inhalants

One can use either tea, essential oils, or a combination as a steam inhalant. Place tea or hot water with essential oils in a container. While still hot, cover the head with a towel, get close to the container and inhale the steam.

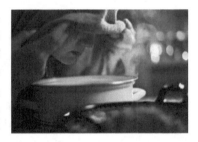

Suppositories

Not used often anymore, people made them for vaginal infections, as well as for laxative effects. Today they are mostly used to administer medicines for those unable to absorb by mouth. Infused herbal oils or powdered herb are mixed with ratio ¾ cocoa butter to oil, and placed into molds, and refrigerated.

Chapter Six
Herbs in Childbearing

Pregnancy Important Warning

Some symptoms ***should not*** be treated at home with herbs.

They need prompt attention from a medical provider.

Signs that need medical attention:

- Continuous bleeding.
- Initial herpes blisters or outbreak.
- Serious pelvic or abdominal pain.
- Continuous serious mid-back pain.
- Hand and face edema.
- Membranes rupture before 37 weeks.
- Regular contractions before 37 weeks.
- Serious headaches, blurred vision, and epigastric pain.
- Fetal movement stopping.

Use intuition, common sense
and knowledgeable resources.

Never hesitate when a child's health and well-being are on the line.

Why Use Herbs in Childbearing?

Since the beginning of time, women have used the power of herbs to safely nurture their body through all cycles of life. Herbs can nourish and strengthen the body to prepare for an easier birth, help recover from postpartum and increase breastmilk. Daily use of nourishing herbs provides excellent, easily assimilated nutrition. Herbs can be effective in reducing the symptoms of common discomforts during pregnancy.

Herbs have been used to increase the strength of contractions during labor, to prevent hemorrhage, to help expel the placenta and promote milk supply. By learning from the traditions of our ancestors, as well as modern science, herbal medicine is a path to healing that empowers individuals and protects the earth.

Are Herbs Safe During Childbearing?

- Many herbs that are unsafe in higher doses are safe in small doses.
- Some are safe during one stage of pregnancy and yet harmful in another.
- List of herbs to avoid in childbearing is extensive, while some are harmful, many have the potential to be dangerous.
- Even if the risk is very small, who wants to take a chance?

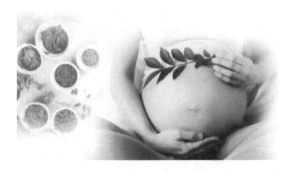

Herb Ratings for Childbearing

Class 1:

- Safe with appropriate use.

Class 2:

- **2a**: For external use only, unless otherwise directed by a professional.
- **2b**: Not for use during pregnancy, unless otherwise directed by a professional with expertise in using the particular substance during pregnancy.
- **2c**: Not for use while breastfeeding, unless otherwise directed by a professional with expertise in using a particular substance while nursing.
- **2d**: Other restrictions according to professional guidance.

Class 3:

- Can be used only under the guidance of a qualified professional.
  (equivalent to requiring a prescription from a physician).

Class 4:

- Insufficient data for classification.
  OR
- X Avoid. Either has been shown to be harmful to mother/fetus or is a toxic plant with no justifiable medical use.

Categories of Herbs to Avoid

- **Abortifacients**: Used to induce abortion or miscarriage.
- **Emmenagogues**: Herbs that promote menstruation.
- **That contains toxic or potentially toxic alkaloids.**
- **That stimulates or mimic hormones or hormonal actions.**
- **Laxatives.**
- **Diuretics.**
  Some herbs can have multiple actions simultaneously.

Abortifacients

These herbs can act as fetotoxins, irritating the uterus to prevent implantation, or induce uterine contractions. Using herbs to induce abortion is unsafe—they often fail, may cause significant side effects, and can lead to complications like bleeding or retained products. In short, it's strongly advised against.

Examples include ashwagandha, cedar, cotton root, elder, juniper, pennyroyal, rue, saffron, scotch broom, spikenard, tansy, thyme, and vetiver.

Emmenagogues

These herbs have varied mechanisms and some, paradoxically, are used in early pregnancy to prevent miscarriage. **Examples include** angel's trumpet, angelica, black cohosh, blue cohosh, catnip, chicory, dill, feverfew, false unicorn root, goldenseal, gotu kola, horehound, hyssop, lovage, motherwort, mugwort, myrrh, parsley, pennyroyal, Roman chamomile, osha, shepherd's purse, tansy, thuja (cedar), trillium, turmeric, valerian, vervain, wild bergamot, wormwood, and yarrow.

Small amounts of basil, rosemary, and turmeric used in cooking are not contraindicated as emmenagogues.

Herbs that Contain Toxic or Potentially Toxic Alkaloids

While effective in treating various illnesses, these herbs can pose risks to a developing fetus. **Examples** include chaparral, comfrey, ephedra, feverfew, ginkgo, ginseng, goldenseal, iris, jimson weed, lobelia, mistletoe, mandrake, mugwort, nutmeg, sassafras, tansy, wintergreen, wild lettuce, white oak, and white willow bark.

Herbs That Stimulate or Mimic Hormones or Actions

While beneficial when appropriately used, misuse of these herbs can lead to hormonal imbalances. **Examples** include angelica, dong quai, evening primrose, fenugreek, ginseng, licorice, red clover, wild yam, and vitex.

Laxatives

Avoid strong herbal laxatives (cathartics and purgatives) during pregnancy because of potential risks such as irritating fetal intestines and inducing premature labor. **Examples** include aloe vera, buckthorn, cascara sagrada, castor oil, goldenseal, Oregon grape root, pokeweed, rhubarb, and senna.

To achieve a laxative effect, consider incorporating fiber and mucilaginous herbs like psyllium, flax, and chia.

Diuretics

Herbs that promote urine flow should generally be avoided during pregnancy due to their potential impact on stressed kidneys. Exceptions include herbs like nettles, which have mild diuretic properties and support kidney function. **Examples include** black cumin, buchu, caraway, cubeb berries, cleavers, dandelion root, corn silk, hops, horse chestnut, horsetail, juniper, parsley, oregano, and urva ursi.

Supportive Herbs in Childbearing Cycle
Nourishing - Preparing - Relieving - Treating

Nourishing

Herbs used often as foods, are generally safe all through pregnancy. They bring specific nutrients that are easier to assimilate than prenatal vitamins. They can gently improve the flow of blood and lymph to the tissue, facilitating optimal nutrition to the cells and removal of cellular waste. **Includes:** alfalfa, borage, burdock, dandelion, ginger root, hibiscus, linden, most mint, nettle, 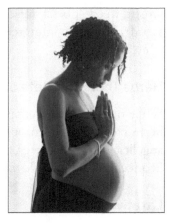 oat straw, peach leaves, raspberry leaf, red clover, rose hips, strawberry leaves, watercress, and yerba buena.

Preparing

Used to prevent problems such as toning the uterus to prepare for a **shorter labor**. Red raspberry leaf is the best preparation herb to use in pregnancy for an easy delivery. Research has shown that eating dates during pregnancy can shorten labor.

Herbs are used only in the last trimester recommended by some sources: black/blue cohosh, cottonwood, motherwort, St. John's wort, and squaw vine (partridge berry).

To avoid postpartum hemorrhage: late in pregnancy or early labor: Alfalfa tablets and probiotics to promote the production of Vitamin K.

Relief during Pregnancy

- **Nausea/Morning Sickness**: Ginger, raspberry leaves, peach leaves, peppermint, linden, nettles, and strawberry leaves.
- **Heartburn**: Marshmallow, slippery elm, peppermint, ginger, fennel, and fenugreek.
- **Headaches**: Lavender (essential oil external), chamomile.
- **Varicosities**: Nettles, oat straw, witch hazel compresses.
- **Stretch Marks**: Calendula, vitamin E, and coconut oil external.
- **Leg Cramps or Muscle Cramps**: Alfalfa and nettle tea.
- **Hemorrhoids**: Yarrow, plantain salve.

Treatment in Pregnancy & Birth

(Use under direction of experienced professional)

- **Threatened miscarriage:** Black haw, false unicorn root, shagari, wild yam.
- **Induce a post-term pregnancy:** castor oil, chamomile.
- **Speed up a slow labor:** Blue/black cohosh, clary sage, motherwort, squaw vine, schisandra, trillium.
- **Rest/pain relief during a long labor:** lobelia, St John's wort, valerian.

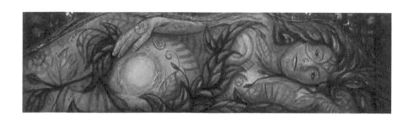

Postpartum Treatments

(Use under direction of experienced professional)

- **Anti-Hemorrhage** (use early): Alfalfa, blue cohosh, motherwort, plantain shepherd's purse, trillium, yarrow.
- **Retained placenta:** Angelica, ground ivy, trillium.
- **Tears and stitches:** Peri rinses with comfrey and sage tea.
- **After-cramps:** Dong quai, cramp bark, raspberry leaves, St. John's wort, and valerian.

Lactation Treatments

- **Herbs to increase milk supply:** Alfalfa, anise seed, blessed thistle, borage, caraway, coriander, fennel seed, dill, goats' rue, milky oat, marshmallow, nettles, fenugreek, shagari, and vitex.
- **Herbs to decrease milk supply:** Corn silk, lemon balm, parsley, sage, and yarrow. Cabbage leaves in the bra for engorgement.

Herbs for Babies

It is not recommended to give herbs to infants by mouth, but baths provide a good way to absorb medicinal properties.

Bath Herbs
- **Colic:** Chamomile, peppermint, fennel, or fenugreek.

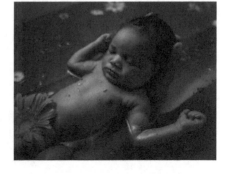

- **Colds and Stuffy Noses:** Eucalyptus, peppermint, sage.
- **Relaxing:** Chamomile, lemon balm, lavender.

Chapter Seven
Eagletree Herbs Recipes

About These Recipes

While I am largely retired from the "business" of Eagletree Herbs, there are a few of these products I still make, sell, barter, and give away. We considered selling the business, but since it was never profitable, that was not an option. A lot of herbal entrepreneurs closely guard their processes or have proprietary blends. Instead, am choosing to give away the recipes we made over the almost fifty years we were in business, hoping the next generation will make some of these products and benefit from the trial and error it took to make them.

Everyone is welcome to use or adapt these recipes for your own use or to sell in your own herbal product business. If any of these recipes help you make a profit, please consider donating to the nonprofit organization, <u>Zaniyan Center</u>. Zaniyan is a Lakota word for a state of health or wholeness. Zaniyan promotes plants for health and a connection to the earth. All the proceeds from this book go to Zaniyan Center.

Our goal was to use organic ingredients, although 100% was not always possible. Assume the following recipes are all organic. We grew and wild-harvested many of our herbs, but never got the yard certified organic, although we grew organically for the twenty-five years I lived in my home.

Not every recipe is here. I started making herbal medicine in the seventies, before personal computers. In the early days, I was not very good at writing recipes down. Some ingredients of the recipes have changed over the years.

Where there is no photo of the product, the label is included. Please keep in mind that you may need to adapt these recipes depending on how you plan to use them, as they are intended for very large quantities. When the recipes changed over the years, the most recent ones are included. These recipes are not exact, there is a certain amount of smelling, testing, and adjusting. Each batch could be a little different, but that is the beauty of homemade.

As we grew and made bigger and bigger batches, we were becoming more of a manufacturer than a herbal medicine maker. Creating a balance between making high quality organic products, ethically and sustainably and being able to make a living, or create a living wage for your employees, is a challenge. While I was never successful, that doesn't mean others are not. There are wonderful herbal businesses out there.

Recipes are listed alphabetically in the categories we used on the Eagletree Herbs website. They are placed under the second word as most of the product names start with "herbal." Many products fall into multiple categories.

While the tincture blends recipes are given, single tinctures are obvious.

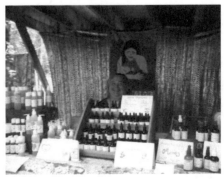

Daphne at the Oregon Country Fair in the 1990s

Categories in this section are:

- Aromatherapy
  - Misters
  - Dream Pillows
  - Bath Salts & Bombs

- Body Care
  - Facial
  - Men's Care

- Culinary Superfoods
  - Chocolate
  - Salts & Seasonings
  - Vinegars
  - Syrups

- First Aid
- Love Products
- Maternity and Baby
- Pest Control
- Salves & Balms
- Syrups and Elixirs (medicinal)
- Smoking Blends
- Teas
- Tinctures

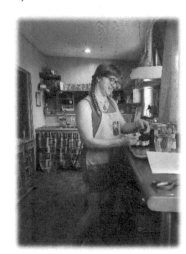

Kelsie started as an intern, was then hired and worked for us for years

Aromatherapy

Some consider that aromatherapy is only with essential oils, but any strong-smelling herbs work.

Breathe Deep Herbal Vapors

Originally made as Baby Vapors, a type of organic "Vicks" in our maternity and baby line, they were so often used by adults we moved them to aromatherapy and changed the name.

Ingredients:

- 5 cups coconut oil.
- ⅛ oz cedar essential oil.
- ⅛ oz sage essential oil.
- ⅛ oz menthol essential oil.
- ⅛ oz spearmint essential oil.
- ⅛ oz wintergreen essential oil.
- ⅛ oz rosemary essential oil.
- ⅛ oz eucalyptus essential oil.
- ⅛ oz lemon eucalyptus essential oil.
- 5 oz of beeswax.

Instructions:

1. Melt coconut oil over low heat.
2. Take off heat and add essential oils and mix.
3. Let cool slightly before pouring.
4. Pour into 2 tins jars.
5. Label.

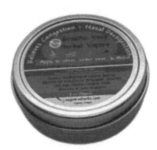

Dead Sea Serenity Bath Salts

Because of the higher mineral content of Dead Sea salts, they are beneficial for certain skin ailments and overall detoxification and moisture replenishment.

Ingredients:

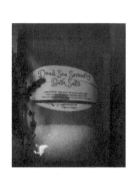

- 4 cups Pure Dead Sea Salts.
- 4 cups Epsom Salts.
- $\frac{1}{8}$ oz lavender essential oil.
- $\frac{1}{8}$ oz ylang ylang essential oil.
- $\frac{1}{8}$ oz orange essential oil.
- $\frac{1}{8}$ oz corn mint essential oil.

Instructions:
1. Measure, combine, and mix all ingredients.
2. Pour into 8 oz bags with cellophane window.
3. Label.

Dream Pillows

Enhance lucid dreaming. Aids restful sleep. Place inside your pillowcase under your head where you can smell and breathe in the power of the herbs while you sleep.

Ingredients:

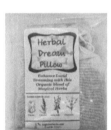

- 8 cups dried chamomile.
- 4 cups dried lavender.
- 6 cups dried mugwort.
- 2 cups dried lemon balm.

Instructions:
1. Measure, combine, and mix all ingredients.
2. Pour into large muslin bags.
3. Place bags 2 oz plastic bags.
4. Label.

Misters

We created signature essential oils blends for our misters and body care products. *Centering Space, Joyfulness, Love Spirit, Clarity and Essential Defender.* They have changed a little over the decades. We mix a large batch of these essential oils and use them for similar products. Under misters, we give the proportions, but subsequently, we refer to them by their signature name. You are welcome to use ours, but creating your own is more fun.

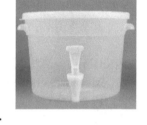

Tip: use a two-gallon dispensing bucket to fill bottles. It is a better two-person job, having someone constantly stirring while filling each bottle to maintain even quantities of essential oils. Or stir after each bottle.
For the end product, colored glass to preserve the quality of the essential oil. Never use plastic bottles for essential oils. It will degrade the plastic, although it can be mixed in a plastic bucket.

Centering Space

Calming and centering. Wonderful for anxiety.

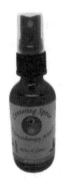

Ingredients:
- ⅛ oz lavender essential oil
- ⅛ oz spearmint essential oil
- 1 gallon distilled water

Instructions:
1. Combine all essential oils to make a blend.
2. Add the essential oil blend to the distilled water.
3. Stir constantly.
4. Bottle in 2 and 4 oz glass bottles with mister tops.
5. Label.

Clarity

To clear away negative energy and attract clear and positive energy.

Ingredients:

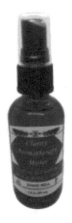

- ⅛ oz cedar essential oil.
- ⅛ oz white sage essential oil.
- 40 drops of sweetgrass essential oil.
- 1 gallon distilled water.

Instructions:
1. Combine all essential oils to make a blend.
2. Add the essential oil blend to the distilled water.
3. Stir constantly.
4. Bottle in 2 and 4 oz glass bottles with mister tops.
5. Label.

Joyfulness

Uplifting and energizing.

Ingredients:

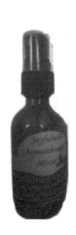

- ⅛ oz orange essential oil
- ⅛ oz lime essential oil
- ⅛ oz tangerine essential oil
- 40 drops ylang ylang essential oil
- 40 drops lavender essential oil
- 1 gallon distilled water

Instructions:

1. Combine all essential oils to make an essential oil blend.
2. Add the essential oil blend to the distilled water.
3. Stir constantly.
4. Bottle in 2 and 4 oz glass bottles with mister tops.
5. Label.

Love Spirit

Attract and enhance love.

Ingredients:

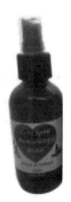

- $\frac{1}{8}$ oz jasmine essential oil.
- 20 drops ginger essential oil
- 40 drops ylang ylang essential oil
- 40 drops rose essential oil
- 20 drops vetiver essential oil
- 1 gallon distilled water

Instructions:

1. Combine all essential oils to make an essential oil blend.
2. Add the essential oil blend to the distilled water.
3. Stir constantly.
4. Bottle in 2 and 4 oz glass bottles with mister tops.
5. Label.

Essential Defender Misters

Our version of "Thieves' Oil." The story of Thieves Oil is from the Middle Ages. Four thieves, who were robbing bubonic plague victims without getting sick, got caught. To get a lighter sentence, they had to reveal their secret formula. Researchers have extensively studied these same herbs and found them to be highly effective against the spread of airborne pathogens. Use when traveling, caring for the sick, and add to the blend to homemade hand sanitizers. You can spray the mister around you or your clothes.

Ingredients:

- 1 gallon distilled water.
- 1 oz clove essential oil.
- 1 oz lemon essential oil
- ½ oz cinnamon essential oil
- ½ oz eucalyptus essential oil
- ¼ oz rosemary essential oil
- ⅛ oz oregano essential oil

Instructions:

1. Combine all essential oils to make an essential oil blend.
2. Add 1 oz of the essential oil blend to 1 gallon of distilled water.
3. Stir constantly.
4. Bottle in 2 and 4 oz glass bottles with mister tops.
5. Label.

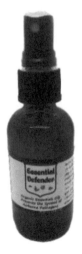

Aromatherapy Roll-ons

Roll-ons are oil-based and last longer than misters. Some, like Essential Defender, apply to face masks, or your nose and upper lip if you are traveling, in crowds, or caring for the sick. Our newest product uses roll-on containers that contain stones that have properties, and we match to each essential oil.

Ingredients:

- 8 oz of fractionated coconut oil.
- ¼ oz of essential oil blend for each type you are making.

Instructions:

1. Add the essential oil blend to oil.
2. Stir often.
3. Pour into 30 ml roll-on bottles.
4. Label.

Body Care

Anti-Fungal Herbal Foot and Body Powder

Best stuff for athlete's foot, just put it in your socks.

Ingredients:

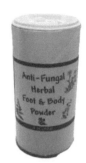

- 4 cups cornstarch.
- 1 cup powdered chamomile.
- 1 cup powdered pau d'arco.
- 1 cup powdered oregano.
- ½ cup powdered spearmint.

Instructions:

1. Measure, combine, and blend all ingredients.
2. Pour into 4 oz cardboard powder shaker containers.
3. Label.

Busy Bee Balm

For dry cracked hands, also good for feet. Beeswax from my daughter Trillium's own bees.

Ingredients:

- 4 cups coconut oil.
- 1 lbs of shea butter.
- 1 cup of infused comfrey oil.
- ½ cup infused calendula oil.
- 5 oz of beeswax.
- 1 tbsp vitamin E.

Instructions:

1. Melt wax and butter over double boiler.
2. Melt coconut oil over low heat.
3. Add wax, butter and mix.
4. Add infused oils and vitamin E.
5. Let cool slightly before pouring.
6. Pour into 2 & 4 oz plastic salve jars.
7. Label.

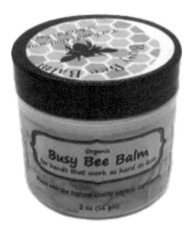

Calendula Hand Lotion

Made during the pandemic for those who had constant handwashing and use of hand sanitizers, which is why it has the "Essential Defender" blend.

Ingredients:

- 4 cups distilled water
- 1.5 cups coconut oil
- 1 cup avocado oil
- ¼ cup shea butter
- 2.5 oz emulsifying wax
- 1 cup calendula infused glycerin
- ¼ cup calendula tincture
- 1 tsp *Essential Defender* essential blend
- ½ tsp of Leucidal (can substitute another preservative)
- ¼ teaspoon grapefruit seed extract

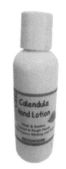

Instructions:

1. Melt wax and butter in a double boiler.
2. Melt coconut oil over low heat.
3. Add wax and butter and mix.
4. Add avocado oil and vitamin E.
5. Put water, essential oils, and glycerin in a sanitized blender.
6. While still warm, pour well mixed oils, wax, and butter in the blender very slowly.
7. Blend well.
8. Pour into 6 oz plastic bottles with pump top.
9. Label.

Calendula Hand Sanitizer with Essential Defender

During the pandemic we wanted to make a more natural hand sanitizer, but still wanted to use the World Health Organization (WHO) formula for safety. We used calendula and our "Essential Defender" essential oil blend.

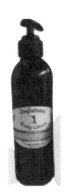

Ingredients:
- 833.3 ml 96% ethanol alcohol.
- 14.5 ml calendula infused glycerin.
- 41.7 ml 3% hydrogen peroxide.
- Enough distilled water to fill the container to 1000 ml.
- ⅛ ounce of Essential Defender blend.

Instructions:
1. Use a 1000 ml container.
2. Combine all ingredients and mix well.
3. After all the other ingredients are added, add just enough distilled water to reach 1000 ml.
4. Pour into 2 oz plastic bottles with flip top lids.
5. Label.

Centering Space & Joyfulness Lotion

A very nice general body lotion.

Ingredients:
- 3 cups coconut oil.
- 5 cups distilled water.
- 2.5 oz emulsifying wax.
- 1 tbsp vitamin E.
- 2 ½ tsp of either essential oil blend.
- ½ tsp of Leucidal (can substitute another preservative).
- 1 tsp rosemary antioxidant.

Instructions:

1. Melt wax in a double boiler.
2. Melt coconut oil over low heat.
3. Add wax and mix.
4. Add vitamin E.
5. Put water and glycerin in a sanitized blender.
6. While still warm, pour well mixed oils, wax, in the blender very slowly. Blend well.
7. Add essential oil last.
8. Let cool slightly before pouring.
9. Pour into 8 oz plastic bottles with a pump top.
10. Label.

Centering Space & Joyfulness Body Butter

The nice thing about body butters is, unlike lotions, they don't need the same level of preservatives and are easier to make.

Ingredients:
- 2 cups coconut oil.
- 1 cup calendula infused olive oil.
- 4 oz mango butter.
- 4 oz shea butter.
- 4 oz mango butter.
- 4 oz cocoa butter.
- 1 tbsp vitamin E.
- 2 tsp lavender essential oil.
- ½ tsp spearmint essential oil.
- 1 tsp rosemary antioxidant.

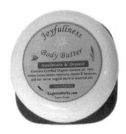

Instructions:
1. Melt butters in a double boiler.
2. Melt coconut oil over low heat.
3. Add butters and mix.
4. Add vitamin E, rosemary and essential oils.
5. Put the whole mix in the refrigerator for one hour.
6. Mix with an electric beater, or preferably a stand mixer.
7. Scoop into 4 oz plastic wide mouth jars.
8. Label.

Earth Tooth Powder

Whitens and protects teeth naturally. Leaves teeth feeling fresh and is completely free of harmful ingredients found in most toothpastes on the market

Ingredients:
- 2 cups bentonite clay
- ½ cup orange peel powder
- ½ cup cinnamon powder
- ¼ cup clove powder
- ⅛ cup myrrh powder
- ¾ cup baking soda
- 2 tbsp stevia powder

Instructions:
1. Measure, combine, and blend all ingredients.
2. Pour into 2 oz glass jars.
3. Label.

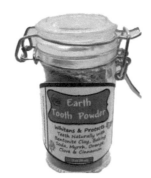

Healing Massage Oil

Especially good for sore and tired muscles, sports massage. The wintergreen is anti-inflammatory, arnica helps prevent bruising, and CBD is for pain.

Ingredients:
- 3 cups comfrey infused olive oil
- 4 cups CBD infused olive oil
- 2 cups arnica infused olive oil
- 2 cups St. John's wort infused olive oil
- 1 cup sweet almond infused olive oil
- 1 tsp wintergreen essential oil 1 tbsp vitamin E
- 1 tsp rosemary antioxidant

Instructions:
1. Measure, combine, and mix all ingredients.
2. Pour into 8 oz plastic bottles with pump tops.
3. Label.

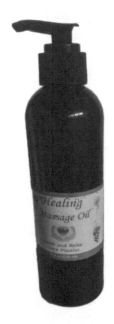

Herbal Deodorant

This stuff is amazing, it works not only as a deodorant, but can prevent heat and chafing rash on thighs.

Ingredients:
- 7 oz beeswax
- ¾ cup chamomile infused oil
- 2 qt. coconut oil
- 2 cups baking soda
- 16 oz cornstarch
- ⅛ ounce lemon essential oil
- 1 tbsp vitamin E oil

Instructions:
1. Melt wax in a double boiler.
2. Melt coconut oil over low heat.
3. Add infused oil.
4. Remove from heat.
5. Add vitamin E.
6. Add essential oil.
7. Pour in baking soda and cornstarch. Blend well.
8. Pour into 2.5 oz plastic deodorant containers.
9. Label.

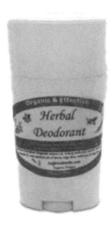

Lotion Candles—Centering Space & Love Spirit

These are so much fun. They are a low temperature candle that turns into a warm lotion. We used our signature essential blends and made two different ones. Fun to demonstrate at events.

Ingredients:
- 75 oz soy wax
- 13 oz coconut oil
- 11.5 oz shea butter
- 3.5 oz cocoa butter
- 8 oz avocado oil
- 8 oz calendula infused olive oil
- ½ tbsp essential oil blend
- 1 tbsp vitamin E oil
- candle wicks

Instructions:
1. Melt butter and wax in a double boiler.
2. Gently melt and mix the oils, wax and butters.
3. Add vitamin E.
4. Let cool slightly before pouring.
5. Remove from heat and then add essential oil.
6. Pour into candle tins.
7. Carefully center wicks with a pair of chopsticks balanced on top of tins until cool.
8. Label.

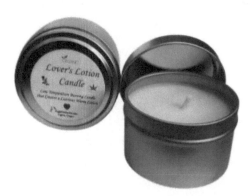

Mango Body Bars

Especially good for legs and hard to reach places.

Ingredients:

- ¾ cup chamomile infused oil
- 4 cups coconut oil
- 2 cups mango butter
- 2 cups shea butter
- 1 cup sweet almond oil
- 7 oz beeswax
- 4 tbsp evening primrose oil
- 1 tbsp vitamin E oil

Instructions:

1. Melt wax in a double boiler.
2. Melt coconut oil over low heat.
3. Mix butter, wax and oils.
4. Remove from heat and add vitamin E.
5. Pour into 2.5 oz plastic deodorant containers.
6. Label.

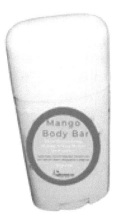

Peppermint Foot Cream

Cooling and absorbing. Great for dry cracked or painful feet.

Ingredients:
- 2 ¾ cup of coconut oil
- ¼ cup of shea butter
- ¼ cup calendula infused oil
- ½ cup of apricot kernel oil
- 2 ½ oz emulsifying wax
- 5 cups distilled water
- peppermint essential oil
- menthol essential oil
- ½ tsp of Leucidal (can substitute another preservative)
- ¼ teaspoon grapefruit seed extract
- 1 tsp rosemary antioxidant
- 1 tbsp vitamin E

Instructions:
1. Melt wax and butter in a double boiler.
2. Melt coconut oil over low heat.
3. Add oils, wax, and mix.
4. Remove from heat and add vitamin E and preservatives.
5. Put water and glycerin in a sanitized blender.
6. While still warm, pour well mixed oils & wax into the blender very slowly. Blend well.
7. Add essential oil last.
8. Let cool slightly before pouring.
9. Pour into 2 & 4 oz plastic jars.
10. Label.

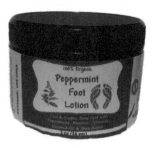

Roots and Locks Hair Oil

As someone with very long hair, I love this.

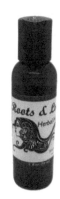

Ingredients:

- 2 cups horsetail infused olive oil
- 2 cups rosemary infused olive oil
- 1 cup sage infused olive oil
- 1 cup nettle infused olive oil
- 1 tbsp vitamin E

Instructions:

1. Mix all oils well.
2. Add vitamin E.
3. Pour into 2oz plastic bottles with a flip top.
4. Label.

Shiny Locks Herbal Hair Rinse

Used after or instead of shampooing.

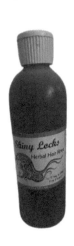

Ingredients:

- 2 cups horsetail infused vinegar
- 2 cups rosemary infused vinegar
- 1 cup lavender infused vinegar
- 1 cup nettle infused vinegar

Instructions:

1. Mix all vinegars well.
2. Pour into 8 oz plastic bottles with a flip top.
3. Label.

Smart Sunscreen

After many years of people at events asking us if we had sunscreen, tried making it. After much research came up with this product. We had both 15 and 30 SPF. Only one problem, the zinc oxide does not absorb well, and it looks a bit like clown makeup if you wear it on your face. Did not end up being so smart. But it was organic.

Ingredients:
- 1 ¾ cup avocado oil.
- 1 lb shea butter.
- 3 oz beeswax.
- 2 oz carrot seed oil
- 1 lb cocoa butter.
- 1 lb mango butter.
- 1 lb coconut oil.
- 7 oz zinc oxide
- 1 tbsp vitamin E

Instructions:
1. Melt wax and butters in a double boiler.
2. Melt coconut oil over low heat.
3. Add oils, wax, and mix.
4. Remove from heat, add vitamin E and the zinc oxide.
5. Let cool slightly before pouring.
6. Pour into 2 oz plastic tubes with flip top cap.
7. Label.

Herbal Toothpaste

Our first attempt at toothpaste. Oil based for tooth pulling. People who tried it loved it, but we could never get it to mix up properly when it cooled off the clay went to the bottom and looked kinda weird.

Ingredients:
- 6 cups coconut oil.
- ½ cup baking soda.
- 3 tsp stevia powder.
- ¼ tsp fine sea salt.
- 20 drops of peppermint essential oil.
- 20 drops spearmint essential oil.
- ½ cup bentonite clay.

Instructions:
1. Gently melt coconut oil.
2. Add and dissolve the baking soda, stevia powder, and bentonite clay.
3. Add the salt in very small increments, and taste as. you go. The salt is extremely variable, too much can really ruin a batch.
4. After adding the correct amount of salt, remove the mixture from heat.
5. Add the essential oils.
6. Let cool slightly before pouring.
7. Pour into 2 oz plastic tubes with flip top cap.
8. Label.

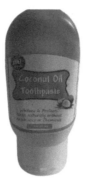

Body Care: Facial

Calendula Facial Cream

Nourishing facial cream that moisturizes, protects, and balances.

Ingredients:

- 1 ½ cups calendula infused olive oil
- ⅔ cup wild rosehip seed oil
- 2 oz beeswax
- ⅔ cup aloe vera gel
- 1 ⅓ cup lemon balm infused glycerin
- 1 ⅔ cup distilled water
- ½ tsp orange essential oil
- 1 tbsp vitamin E oil
- ½ tsp of Leucidal or other preservative
- ¼ teaspoon grapefruit seed extract
- ¼ tsp rosemary antioxidant

Instructions:

1. Melt wax in a double boiler.
2. Melt coconut oil over low heat.
3. Add wax and oil and mix.
4. Put water and infused glycerin in a sanitized blender.
5. While still warm, pour well mixed oils, wax, in the blender very slowly. Blend well.
6. Add essential oil, vitamin E and preservatives last.
7. Let cool slightly before pouring.
8. Pour into ½ oz glass jars.
9. Label.

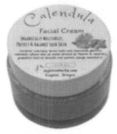

Charcoal Sea Scrub

The activated charcoal will bind to any toxins you have on your skin, and the salt will scrub off dead skin cells. The only problem was that you had to use it in the shower otherwise the black was hard to get off.

Ingredients:
- 4 cups activated charcoal.
- 2 cups coconut oil.
- ½ cup shea butter.
- ⅛ ounce ylang ylang essential oil.
- ⅛ ounce spearmint essential oils
- ⅛ ounce lavender essential oils
- Vitamin E

Instructions:
1. Melt butter in a double boiler.
2. Melt coconut oil over low heat.
3. Add butter and oil and mix.
4. Remove from heat.
5. Mix in the charcoal slowly
6. Add essential oil and vitamin E.
10. Pour into 4 oz clear glass jars.
11. Label.

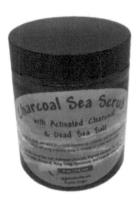

Herbal Facial Serum

Very light absorbing serum with calendula at a fraction of the cost of similar products.

Ingredients:
- 24 oz kukui nut oil
- 8 oz rosehip seed oil
- 5 oz apricot seed oil
- 1 1/3 cup calendula infused glycerin
- ½ tsp sweet orange essential oil
- ¼ tsp rosemary antioxidant
- 1 tbsp vitamin E

Instructions:
1. Mix all oils and glycerin well.
2. Melt coconut oil over low heat.
3. Add wax and oil and mix.
4. Add essential oil, vitamin E and preservatives.
5. Pour into 1oz glass bottles with treatment pump top.
6. Label.

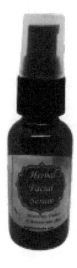

Herbal Facial Toner

An astringent toner that goes with all facial care. We bought the expensive organic witch hazel from Mountain Rose, but you can use the witch hazel from the drug store as well.

Ingredients:
- 2 quarts witch hazel
- ¾ cup dried lemon balm, ¼ cup fresh lemon balm
- ¾ cup dried sage, ¼ cup fresh sage
- ¾ cup dried rosemary, ¼ cup fresh rosemary
- ¼ tsp lavender essential oil

Instructions:
1. In a gallon jar, place all herbs, cover with witch hazel.
2. Infuse one month in a dark place with periodic shaking.
3. Strain.
4. Pour into 2 oz bottles with a flip top.
5. Label.

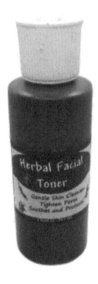

Garden Goddess Herbal Clay Mask
Great for oily skin and acne prone areas

Ingredients:
- 1 cup bentonite clay
- 1 cup French green clay
- 1 cup chamomile powder
- ½ cup rose petal powder
- ½ cup rosemary powder

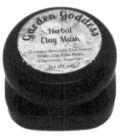

Instructions:
1. Mix all powders well.
2. Pour into 3 oz containers.
3. Label.

Licorice Lightening Cream
Licorice is supposed to be good for age spots. It did not miraculously get rid of mine, but it is a nice face cream.

Ingredients:
- 1.5 cup calendula infused oil
- 2/3 cup coconut oil
- 2 oz emulsifying wax

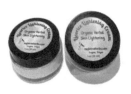

- 1 1/3 cup licorice infused glycerin
- 1 2/3 cup distilled water
- 1 tsp lavender essential oil
- 1 tsp tangerine essential oil
- 1 tsp ylang ylang essential oil
- 1 tbsp vitamin E oil
- ½ tsp of Leucidal or other preservative
- ¼ tsp grapefruit seed extract
- ¼ tsp rosemary antioxidant

Instructions:

1. Melt wax in a double boiler.
2. Melt coconut oil over low heat.
3. Add wax and oil and mix.
4. Add infused glycerin.
5. Add vitamin E.
6. Put water and glycerin in a sanitized blender.
7. While still warm, pour well mixed oils, wax, in the blender very slowly. Blend well.
8. Add essential oil and preservatives last.
9. Let cool slightly before pouring.
10. Bottle in ½ oz glass jars.
11. Label.

Lip Balm

A festival staple. A few years ago, we tried to make one with a bit of lip color with beet and hibiscus powder, but it did not go well.

Ingredients:

- 3 cups coconut oil
- 1 cup apricot kernel oil
- 1 cup shea butter
- 1 cup mango butter
- 8 oz beeswax
- 40 ml hemp oil
- ⅛ oz sweet orange essential oil
- 1 tbsp vitamin E

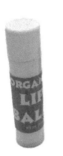

Instructions:

1. Melt wax and butters in a double boiler.
2. Melt coconut oil over low heat.
3. Add oils, wax and mix.
4. Remove from heat and add vitamin E.
5. Let cool slightly before pouring.
6. Pour into 5.5 ml lip balm tubes.
7. Label.

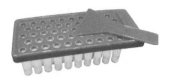

Handy lip balm filling tray

Rose Sugar Scrub

This scrub is both exfoliative and moisturizing. We made it with calendula oil, but could be made with calendula glycerin instead.

Ingredients:

- 2 ½ cups rose petals
- 2 1/4 cups calendula infused oil
- 2 lb organic sugar
- 1/4 tsp lavender essential oil

Instructions:

1. Measure and blend all ingredients.
2. Pour into wide mouth 4 oz jars.
3. Label.

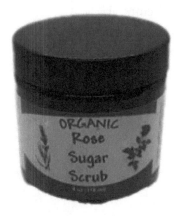

Body Care: Men's Line

Another of Trillium's products. Starts with Bright Morning and ends with Rough Night.

Bright Morning Aftershave

Ingredients:

- 1 qt sage infused witch hazel
- 1qt rosemary infused witch hazel
- 16 fl. oz plain witch hazel
- ½ cup calendula infused glycerin
- 1 tsp sandalwood essential oil
- ⅛ tsp myrrh & cedar essential oil
- ½ tsp bay essential oil

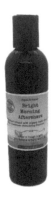

Instructions:
1. Mix and blend well.
2. Pour into 8 oz bottles with flip top lids.
3. Label.

Bright Morning Shaving Soap

Ingredients:

- 4 cups coconut oil
- 4 cups African black soap liquid
- 1 cup cocoa butter
- ½ cup calendula infused olive oil
- 3 tbsp emulsifying wax
- 2 tbsp bentonite clay
- ¼ cup calendula infused glycerin
- ⅛ ounce sandalwood, bay, amber essential oils
- 2 tbsp grapefruit seed extract
- 1 tbsp vitamin E

Instructions:
1. Melt wax and butter in a double boiler.
2. Add oils, wax and mix.
3. Remove from heat, add vitamin E and essential oils.
4. Blend well with immersion blender.
5. Let cool slightly before pouring.
6. Pour into 4 oz tins.
7. Label.

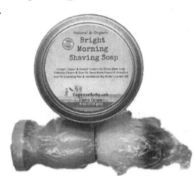

Included a free shaving brush.

Rough Night Beard Oil

Ingredients:
- 24 oz sweet almond oil
- 16 oz jojoba oil
- 4 oz argon oil
- ½ tsp blend of sandalwood, bay, & amber essential oils
- ¼ tsp rosemary antioxidant
- 1 tbsp vitamin E

Instructions:
1. Mix all oils well.
2. Add essential oil, vitamin E and preservatives.
3. Pour into 2 oz bottles with flip top or treatment pump.
4. Label.

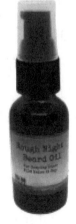

Rough Night Mustache Wax

Ingredients:
- 24 oz sweet almond oil
- 16 oz jojoba oil
- 4 oz argon oil
- ½ tsp blend of sandalwood, bay, & amber essential oils
- ¼ tsp rosemary antioxidant
- 1 tbsp vitamin E

Instructions:
1. Melt wax and butter in a double boiler.
2. Add oils, wax and mix.
3. Remove from heat, add vitamin E, rosemary, and essential oils.
4. Let cool slightly before pouring.
5. Pour into 2 oz tins.
6. Label.

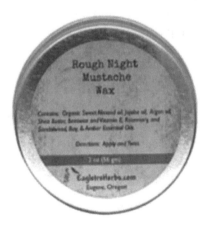

Culinary Superfoods

Chocolate

Herb Chocolates (not that kind)
We only made chocolates for a year or two, when we were doing farmer's markets on a weekly basis. Only pictures of labels.

Lavender Chocolates
Ingredients:

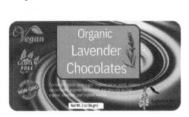

- 3 lbs coconut oil
- 3 lbs sugar
- 3 lbs coco nibs
- 3 oz lavender

Instructions:
1. Simmer the lavender in oil over very low heat for one hour.
2. Strain the oil and add coco nibs until melted.
3. Add the sugar while warm, allowing it to melt completely.
4. Combine oil, cocoa, and sugar.
5. Pour into molds and cool in the fridge.
6. Wrap in three packs in cellophane bags.
7. Label.

Inner Glow Chocolates
Ingredients:

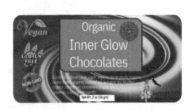

- 3 lbs coconut oil
- 3 lbs organic sugar
- ½ cup cinnamon
- ½ cup ginger
- 1 oz cardamom powder
- 2 tbsp cayenne powder

Instructions:
1. Melt coconut oil over very low heat for one hour.
2. Add the sugar while warm, allowing it to melt completely.
3. Mix in the powdered herbs.
4. Pour into molds and cool in the fridge.
5. Wrap in three packs in cellophane bags.
6. Label.

Inner Glow Cocoa Mix

Hot cocoa with a little kick. Very popular for Christmas gifts. People added the milk of their choice.

Ingredients:
- 6 lbs organic cocoa powder (sweet ground chocolate)
- 5 lbs organic sugar
- 1.5 cups cinnamon powder
- 1 oz cardamom powder
- 1 cup ginger powder
- 2 tbsp cayenne powder

Instructions:
1. Measure, combine, and blend all ingredients.
2. Pour into clear glass 12oz mugs with handle.
3. Label.

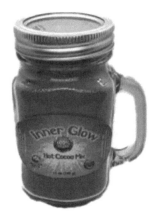

Herbal Honeys
We made three types, all made the same way, but with different herbs.

Ingredients:
- A little less than 1 gallon of local raw honey
- 4 cups dried lavender **or** dried spearmint

For Inner Glow:
- 1 cup cinnamon chips
- 1 cup dried ginger root
- ½ cup cracked cardamon pods
- ½ cup whole black peppercorn
- ½ cup whole chili peppers

Instructions:
1. Make infused honeys according to the instructions for infused oils.
2. Stain the herbs out using a canning funnel and a large pestle-like tool. (There may be better methods)
3. Pour strained honey into 2 and 4 oz honey jars.
4. The left over herbs can be used as an electuary for tea.
5. Label.

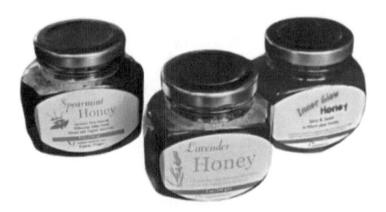

Salts & Superfood Seasonings

Kale Sprinkles

Our most commercially successful product, people still track me down and ask for it. It is both a seasoning and a superfood supplement. You can add it to almost any savory food. If anyone wants to make it commercially, contact me, as I still own the trademark, but will give it someone able to make it and donate a little to my nonprofit.

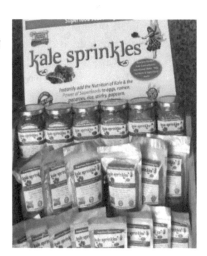

Ingredients:

- 3 lb of dried kale
- 3 lb of nutritional yeast
- 1 lb nettle powder
- 0.75 lb of onion granules
- 0.5 lb of turmeric
- 0.25 lb of onion powder
- 0.25 lb of parsley
- 1.25 lb of garlic granules
- 0.25 lb of kelp
- 0.25 lb of oregano
- 3 tablespoons of cumin

For Kaliente Blend add *per one gallon of Festival blend.
- 15 tablespoons of chili flakes,
  ½ tablespoon of cayenne powder.

Instructions:

1. Measure, combine, and blend all the powders in a five-gallon bucket.
2. Add the kale and nettles.
3. Mix well, we used an electric drill and a paint stirrer.
4. Put into various size containers. Include the ½ oz trial size.
5. Label.

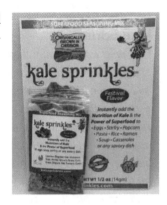

Italiano Herb Salt

These are a nice way to preserve fresh herbs.

Ingredients:

- 2 cups fresh basil that has been drying for two days
- 1 1/2 cups fresh oregano
- 1 1/2 cups fresh thyme
- 1 cup minced garlic
- 6 cups Celtic Sea salt

Instructions:

1. Measure, combine, and blend all ingredients in a food processor.
2. Pour into 2-ounce jars.
3. Label.

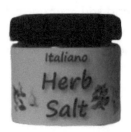

Mushroom Salt

Adds an umami flavor. These mushrooms are really good for you, but it is 50% salt, so people eat little of it. The small packets sold for only $2.00, and they made nice stockings stuffers and impulse buys.

Ingredients:

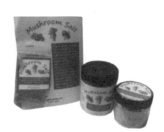

- 3 cups lobster mushrooms
- 3 cups maitake mushrooms
- 6 cups shitake mushrooms
- 12 cups Celtic Sea salt

Instructions:

1. Measure, combine, and blend all ingredients in a food processor.
2. Pour into 2- & 4-ounce jars and ½ ounce Ziplock bags.
3. Label.

Scarborough Fair Salt

The younger generation won't remember, Simon and Garfunkel popularized a very old song about going to the market for these four herbs.

Ingredients:

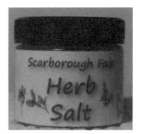

- 1 cup dried parsley
- 1 cup dried sage
- 1 cup dried rosemary
- 1 cup dried thyme
- 4 cups Celtic Sea salt

Instructions:

1. Mix herbs and salt very well.
2. Pour into 1 ounce glass wide mouth jars.
3. Label.

Scarborough Fair Seasoning Blend

Similar in flavor to Herbs de Provence. This was the easiest product to make. Grew the herbs in the front yard, and mix, dry and package.

Ingredients:
- 2 cups dried parsley
- 2 cups dried sage
- 2 cups dried rosemary
- 2 cups dried thyme

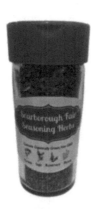

Instructions:
1. Mix herbs very well.
2. Pour into 2 oz glass seasoning jars.
3. Label.

Volcano Salt

Made with red Alaea salt which is processed with the legendary red clay rich in iron oxides found only in Hawaii. Black Lava salt is infused with activated charcoal. We add cayenne for the kick. Picture doesn't show it, but we layered the red salt, then black. It looked cool.

Ingredients:
- 4 cups Alaea salt
- 4 cups black lava salt
- 1 tablespoon cayenne pepper

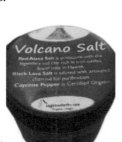

Instructions:
1. Mix the cayenne with the Alaea salt very well.
2. Pour a small amount of the red salt, then meticulously layer the black salt until the 2-ounce jar is filled.
3. Label.
4. Try not to jostle on the way to the market.

Syrups–Culinary

Lavender Syrup

A lovely syrup, but only made a short time because without canning the syrups needed refrigeration or it molded. We did not want to use alcohol preservatives.

Ingredients:

- 4 cups dried lavender. Can substitute roses
- 1 gallon distilled water
- 2 gallons of sugar (really)

Instructions:

1. Boil the water, take off heat when it comes to a rolling boil.
2. Add the dried lavender, cover and let sit for 20 minutes.
3. Strain well and add back into a large enough pot.
4. Add the sugar, over a very low heat, melt sugar.
5. Remove from heat.
6. Pour into 10-ounce sauce bottles.
7. Label.

Mojito Mint Mixer

One of my favorite products. I am not much of a drinker, so I never added more rum, but most people did. Add carbonated water and rum to taste.

Ingredients:

- 4 cups dried mojito mint. Can substitute spearmint
- 1 gallon distilled or filtered water
- 2 gallons of sugar (really)
- 16 fl. oz lime juice
- 1 cup of light rum as a preservative

Instructions:

1. Boil the water, take off heat when it comes to a rolling boil.
2. Add the dried mint, cover and let sit for 20 minutes. Strain well and add back into a large enough pot.Add the sugar, over a very low heat, melt sugar. Remove from heat.
3. Add the lime juice, rum and mix well.
4. Pour into 10-ounce sauce bottles.
5. Label.

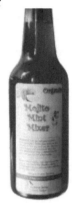

Vinegars

Digestive Vinegar

Be sure to make this with raw organic vinegar with the "mother."

Ingredients:
- 1 cup marshmallow infused vinegar
- 1 cup yellow dock infused vinegar
- 1 cup dandelion infused vinegar
- ½ cup lemon balm infused vinegar
- ½ cup ginger infused vinegar

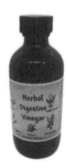

Instructions:
1. Mix all vinegars together well.
2. Pour into 4 oz glass bottles.
3. Label.

Dragon's Breath Cider

Trillium's Fire Cider Recipe, wonderful product. Going to keep making it just for us.

Ingredients:

- 1 cup rosemary infused vinegar
- 2 cups cardamon infused vinegar
- ½ cup Thai chili infused vinegar
- 4 cups raw apple cider vinegar
- 6 ½ cups ginger infused vinegar
- ¼ cup ground pepper vinegar
- 2 cups cayenne infused vinegar
- 1 qt honey

Instructions:

1. Heat slowly over low heat.
2. Dissolve and melt the honey.
3. Blend well.
4. Pour into 10 oz glass sauce bottles.
5. Place one dry Thai chili in each bottle.
6. Label.

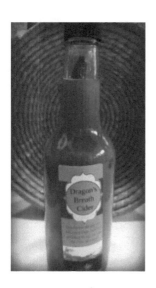

Tonigrette

The best for the immune system, if I take it at the earliest signs, I don't get sick. Everyone around me got Covid, but I never did. Be sure to make with organic vinegar with the "mother."

Ingredients:

- 11 cups nettles infused vinegar
- 8 cups oregano infused vinegar
- 8 cups garlic infused vinegar
- ½ cup rosemary infused vinegar
- ¼ cup cayenne infused vinegar

Instructions:

1. Mix strained vinegars well.
2. Pour into 10 oz glass sauce bottles.
3. Place a spring of fresh rosemary inside.
4. Label.

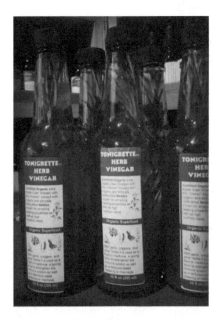

First Aid

Herbal First Kit

This was a great product that did not sell as well as I had hoped. Perfect for travel or camping as well as home use.

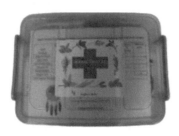 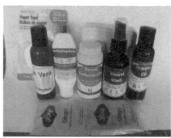

Contained:

- Herbal Wound Wash
- Herbalsporin
- Bentonite clay with calendula
- Aloe Vera gel infused with calendula
- Trauma Oil

Also included: a box of bandages, tape, ginger tea bag, honey stick, charcoal tablets, and a card with emergency first aid and CPR instructions.

Bentonite Clay with Calendula

It is good poison oak and bleeding cuts.

Ingredients:

- 4 cups bentonite clay
- 1 cup calendula powder

Instructions:

1. Mix all powders well.
2. Pour into 4 oz cardboard shaker containers.
3. Label.

Wound Wash
Spray antiseptic, also used for poison oak.

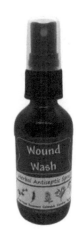

Ingredients:
- 2 cups comfrey infused witch hazel
- 2 cups rosemary infused witch hazel
- 2 cups yarrow infused witch hazel
- 2 cups calendula infused witch hazel

Instructions:
1. Mix and blend well.
2. Pour into 2 and 4 oz bottles with spray tops.
3. Label.

Love Products

Aphrodite Massage Oil
Massage oil for lovers. Oil-based products should not be used with condoms. We got tired of giving that warning out at events, and consequently made our organic Lover's Lube.

Ingredients:
- 4 cups rose petal infused sunflower oil
- 4 cups damiana infused sunflower oil
- 4 cups CBD infused olive oil
- 4 cup sweet almond oil
- ⅛ oz jasmine essential oil.
- 20 drops ginger essential oil
- 40 drops ylang ylang essential oil
- 40 drops rose essential oil
- 20 drops vetiver essential oil
- 1 tbsp vitamin E
- 1 tsp rosemary antioxidant

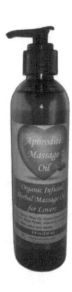

Instructions:

1. Measure, combine, and mix all ingredients.
2. Pour into 8 oz red plastic bottles with pump tops.
3. Label.

Date Night Sauce

Aphrodisiac herbs in a chocolate sauce. Really.

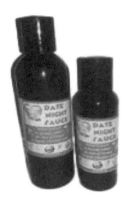

Ingredients:
- 8 cups distilled water.
- ½ cup matcha alcohol tincture.
- ½ cup yohimbe alcohol tincture.
- 1 cup horny goat weed glycerin.
- 2 cups damiana glycerin.
- 2 cups muira puama glycerin.
- 1 cup ashwagandha glycerin.
- 16 cups organic sugar.
- 10 cup cocoa powder.

Instructions:
1. Slowly dissolve the sugar into the water.
2. Add the cocoa powder.
3. Remove from heat and add the glycerin.
4. Add the tinctures.
5. Mix well.
6. Pour into 2 & 4 red plastic bottles with flip tops.
7. Label.

Lovers Lube

Today there are lots of organic lube options, back then we were the only one I knew about.

Ingredients:

- 8 cups distilled water.
- 1 ½ cups damiana glycerin.
- 2 tbsp guar gum.
- ½ tsp of Leucidal (can substitute another preservative).

Instructions:

1. Mix water and glycerin in a blender.
8. Add the preservative.
9. Add the guar gum.
10. Mix well.
11. Pour into 2 & 4 oz plastic bottles with flip tops.
    (we had heart-shaped glass bottles to start)
12. Label.

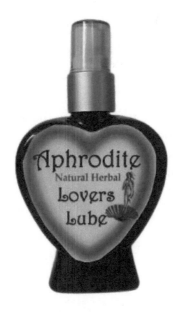

Maternity and Baby

Baby Bath Herbs

Ingredients:

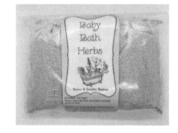

- 2 cups dried lemon balm
- 2 cups dried chamomile
- 2 cups dried lavender
- 1 cup dried spearmint

Instructions:
1. Mix all herbs well.
2. Put into large muslin bags. Put three bags in a Ziplock or cellophane bag.
3. Label.

Baby Bottom Salve

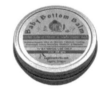

It really works.

Ingredients:
- 1 cups chamomile infused oil
- 1 cups calendula infused oil
- ½ cup comfrey infused oil
- ½ cup cleavers infused oil
- 3 oz beeswax
- 1 tbsp vitamin E

Instructions:
1. Melt wax in a double boiler.
2. Add oils, heat over low heat until well mixed.
3. Remove from heat, add vitamin E.
4. Let cool slightly before pouring.
5. Pour into 1 oz tins.
6. Label.

Belly Balm

One of our very first products, before we were even Eagletree Herbs.

Ingredients:

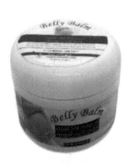

- 32 oz coconut oil
- 8 oz calendula infused olive oil
- 4 oz cocoa butter
- 4 oz mango butter
- 4 oz beeswax
- 1 tbsp vitamin E

Instructions:

1. Melt wax and butter in a double boiler.
2. Add oils, heat over low heat until well mixed.
3. Remove from heat, add vitamin E.
4. Let cool slightly before pouring.
5. Pour into 4 oz wide mouth plastic jars.
6. Label.

Chapless Cheekies

Used for both babies and adults with heat rashes. For years, we powdered our own herbs in a food processor, buying them pre-powdered is much easier.

Ingredients:

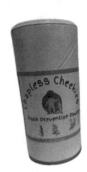

- 1 cup lavender powder
- 1 cup calendula powder
- 1 cup chamomile powder
- 1 lb arrowroot
- 1 lb bentonite clay

Instructions:

1. Mix all powders well.
2. Pour into 4 oz cardboard shaker containers.
3. Label.

Nipple Balm

Sore nipples can be a big problem, this balm helps, but also consult professionals about positioning.

Ingredients:
- 3 oz beeswax
- 1 cup shea butter
- 1 cup coconut oil
- 1 lb lanolin (anhydrous)
- 1 cup infused calendula oil
- 1 cup infused yarrow oil
- 1 tbsp vitamin E

Instructions:
1. Melt wax and butter in a double boiler.
2. Add to coconut oil and heat over low heat until well mixed.
3. Add infused oil and lanolin.
4. Remove from heat, add vitamin E.
5. Let cool slightly before pouring.
6. Pour into ½ oz jars.
7. Label.

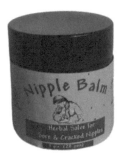

Pregnancy Tea

Safe for all stages of pregnancy, after 30 years of midwifery, I believe it works.

Ingredients:

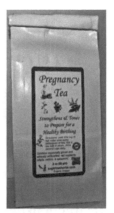

- 4 cups cup dried red raspberry leaf
- 4 cups dried nettle leaf
- 3 cups alfalfa leaf
- 1 cup spearmint leaf

Instructions:
1. Mix all herbs well.
2. Pour into 2 oz bags.
3. Label.

Nursing Mother Tea

Some good evidence supports these herbs along with other methods a lactation professional can help with.

Ingredients:

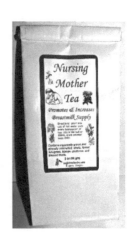

- 2 cups dried borage
- 2 cups dried blessed thistle
- 2 cups alfalfa leaf
- 1 cup goat's rue
- ½ cup fennel
- ½ cup fenugreek

Instructions:
1. Mix all herbs well.
2. Pour into 2 oz bags.
3. Label.

Pest Control

Herbal Flea Powder

Safe for pets even if they lick it, put it on them and in their bedding.

Ingredients:
- 24 cups diatomaceous earth
- 4 cups powdered pennyroyal
- 4 cups powdered eucalyptus
- 1 cup powdered oregano
- 1/2 cup powdered rosemary

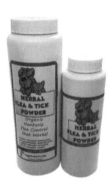

Instructions:
1. Mix everything well.
2. Pour into 2 oz and 4 oz white powder shaker containers.
3. Label.

Mosquidaddle Mosquito Repellent

This has been selling at the Oregon Country Fair beginning in 1977, has supported our booth since. There are terrible mosquitos there and thousands of fair goers for forty-seven years can't be wrong when they say it is the best mosquito repellent, and works better than DEET or OFF. It not only works to prevent bites, but if you already have bites, it can soothe the itch.

A 2024 study found that catnip essential oil diluted to 2% was able to repel over 70% of mosquitoes for up to four hours. Another study found that catnip essential oil at a dosage of 20 mg repelled 96% of stable flies and 79% of houseflies.

The essential oil in catnip that gives it its odor, nepetalactone, may be up to ten times more effective at repelling mosquitoes than DEET.

The oil directly on the skin is the most effective and needs to be reapplied if you no longer smell it. After decades of people asking us to make a water-based spray we finally gave in and made a spray, but we also have to warn people it does not work as well.

We only make it once a year, and we make 5-10 gallons a year. The formula has changed a little over the years, as well as the carrier oil used. I am not listing the exact recipe, because there is not one. It is a bit of a pour and sniff method. Or magic Every year I say I am going to measure it, and between one thing and another it never happens. My children and grandchildren know how to make it.

Contains: organic sunflower oil, and the essential oils of citronella, eucalyptus, litsea, geranium, catnip, camphor, cinnamon, & pennyroyal.

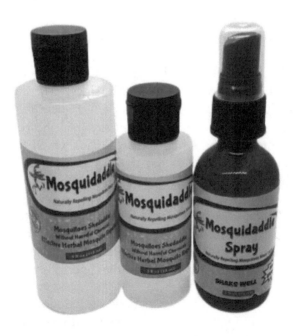

Words to the song my sister Kahish wrote about Mosquidaddle. It was so fun singing it with her and the kids. I hope to find the video of her singing it and put it on my YouTube channel.

Mosquidaddle Song

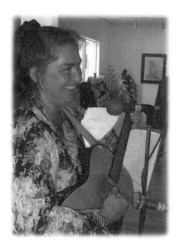

I was at the country fair

Having lots of fun

When a pesky mosquito

Bit me on my bun

It was really annoying

I wanted it to leave

Mosquitos must skedaddle

I need some relief

: M o s q u i t o s must, they must they must skedaddle

They must, they must, they must skedaddle

I needed something natural

Something without Deet

I need my brain to function

It operates my feet

I discovered Mosquidaddle at fair booth 44

It's natural, it's safe and

I'm not bothered anymore

M o s q u i t o s must, they must they must skedaddle

They must, they must, they must skedaddle

I was ready to travel where mosquitoes love to hang

I wanted to be peaceful, because that is my thang

Before I got my bearings, assumed the pose to meditate

It was a drive by biting, i was the dinner plate

> **Chorus:** *mosquitos must, they must they must skedaddle (3)*
> *they must skedaddle now!*

Skitters and no see ums, got me good at dinner time

I slathered Mosquidaddle, to avoid West Nile and Lyme

Those diseases can be fatal, from just a little bite

So I use Mosquidaddle before I say goodnight

> **Chorus:** *mosquitos must, they must they must skedaddle (3)*
> *they must skedaddle now!*

I was scratching, scratching, scratching, the mosquitoes bites did itch,

I know it's not the best thing, but itching is a bitch

Mosquidaddle also soothes, when discomfort does ignite

It calmed the twitches in my britches from my big mosquito bite

> **Chorus:** *mosquitos must, they must they must skedaddle (3)*
> *they must skedaddle now!*

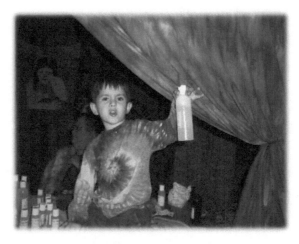

Grandson Zane selling Mosquidaddle 2001

Nit Git Lice Kit

I thought this would be a huge seller, few organic lice treatments were available at the time. Spent a tremendous amount of time in research and sourcing materials. Came up with a great kit, which included a lice comb and a shower cap, and a handout giving a step-by-step effective treatment regime. Did not sell very many kits. But including the information from the accompanying handout because I worked so dang hard on it.

Nit Git Spray

Ingredients:
- 1 gallon apple cider vinegar
- ⅛ oz tea tree essential oil
- ⅛ oz lemon essential oil
- ⅛ oz lavender essential oil
- ⅛ oz neem essential oil

Instructions:
1. Mix everything well.
2. Pour into a 4 oz glass spray bottle.
3. Label.

Nit Git Rub

Ingredients:
- 4 cups coconut oil
- 4 oz beeswax
- 2 cups diatomaceous earth
- 1 tbsp vitamin E

Instructions:
1. Melt wax and butter in a double boiler.
2. Add to coconut oil and heat over low heat until well mixed.
3. Remove from heat, add essential oils and vitamin E.
4. Let cool slightly before pouring.
5. Pour into 4 oz plastic wide mouth jars.
6. Label.

Included with the kit are the instructions.

Git Rid of Lice for Good with Nit Git

Step 1—Spray & Comb

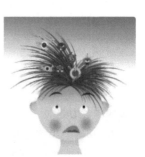

- Spray the hair with Nit Git 100% Organic Vinegar Spray with Essential Oils. This kills most of the lice and unsticks the glue from the nits.
- Rinse with any hair conditioner.
- Comb hair while wet using the fine-toothed nit comb in your kit. Separate the hair in small sections that are about 1 inch by ½ inch, starting at the scalp and ending with the tip. Comb the entire length of wet and lubricated hair. Make sure to clean the comb with a tissue and some hot water after you've combed each section. Use good light, or even a magnifying glass. Pin up sections of the hair you've already combed to ensure that you get the entire scalp.

Step 2 – Rub to Kill & Smother the Little Suckers

- Apply Nit Git 100% Organic Oil Rub. Containing both food grade diatomaceous earth (DE) and essential oils, any of the little buggers left alive will not be for much longer. Just to make totally sure, apply enough to smother them. You may need to heat the oil some to get it all out, but do not microwave.
- Cover the entire head, then apply the shower cap in your kit, then wrap this with a towel and leave on overnight or at least 8 hours.

Step 3—Shampoo

- In the morning, thoroughly shampoo hair with any shampoo of your choice. You may need to do it twice to get all the DE out. Use a good conditioner, white helps you see them.

Step 4—Spray and Comb

- Repeat step one, spray hair and comb again. All of the lice and 99% of the nits are probably dead, but just in case, because this is such a pain in the rear end, you only want to do this once

Step 5—Prevent Reinfection

- Clean household items the affected person has used within the past three days. Wash bedding, stuffed animals, and clothing in hot and soapy water. The water should be at least 130 degrees Fahrenheit. Dry items at a high heat
- Wash hair care items such as combs, brushes, and accessories in hot, soapy water. Soak the items in water that is at least 130 degrees Fahrenheit for five to ten minutes
- Seal any items that you cannot clean or wash in a plastic bag for two weeks to deprive the lice and nits of air. Or put in a freezer for 24 hours
- Vacuum your floors and any upholstered furniture
- Inspect vigilantly for a couple of weeks and inspect the head often for evidence of any lice or their nits. Nits hatch seven to eleven days after being laid, so check the daily scalp for at least two weeks after treatment and then every regularly thereafter to detect any reinfestation
- Use Nit Git Sp ray to prevent them from coming back

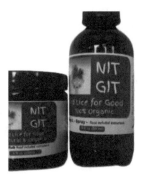

Salves and Balms

Green Relief

Another best seller I will keep making. This works much better than other CBD pain topicals because of quality homegrown ingredients, and the wintergreen, which has salicylic acid like aspirin and is anti-inflammatory as well as cooling.

Ingredients:

- 12 cups CBD oil
- 12 cups olive oil
- 6 cups comfrey infused olive oil
- 2 cups St. John's wort infused olive oil
- 2 cups arnica infused olive oil
- 34 oz beeswax
- 3 oz menthol crystals
- 1 tbsp cajaput essential oil
- 1 oz wintergreen essential oil
- ½ oz peppermint essential oil
- ½ oz spearmint
- 4 tbsp vitamin E

Instructions:

1. Melt wax in a double boiler.
2. Add to oils and heat over low heat until well mixed.
3. Remove from heat, add vitamin E and essential oils.
4. Let cool slightly before pouring.
5. Pour into 2 and 4 oz green plastic jars.
6. Label.

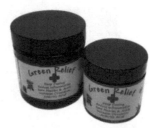

Herbalsporin

Our first decade or two, this was called Boo Boo Salve.

Ingredients:

- 2 cups comfrey infused olive oil
- 2 cups plantain infused olive oil
- 2 cups yarrow infused olive oil
- 2 cups cleavers infused olive oil
- 8 oz beeswax
- 1 tbsp vitamin E

Instructions:

1. Melt wax in a double boiler.
2. Add to oils and heat over low heat until well mixed.
3. Remove from heat, add vitamin E.
4. Let cool slightly before pouring.
5. Pour into ½ oz glass jars.
6. Label.

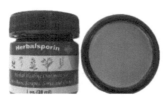

Lizard Balm

Our remedy for eczema balm or dry, itchy, scaly skin.

Ingredients:

- 1 cup cleavers infused olive oil
- 1 cup comfrey infused olive oil
- 1 cup calendula infused olive oil
- 1 cup usnea infused olive oil
- 1/2 cup shea butter
- 1/4 cup jojoba oil
- 4 oz beeswax
- 1 tbsp vitamin E

Instructions:

1. Melt butter and wax in a double boiler.
2. Mix oils.
3. Add wax and butter, mix well.
4. Add vitamin E.
5. Let cool slightly before pouring.
6. Pour into 1 oz plastic salve jars.
7. Label.

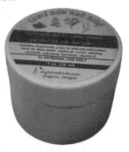

Red Relief

More of a liniment than a balm, same base as Green Relief, but in a roll-on applicator with warming essential oils and a little hot pepper inside.

Ingredients:

- ½ gallon CBD oil
- 3 cups comfrey infused olive oil
- 1 cup St. John's wort infused olive oil
- 3 cups arnica infused olive oil
- 1 cup cayenne infused olive oil
- 1 oz cajeput essential oil
- 40 drops cinnamon leaf essential oil
- 2 tbsp vitamin E

Instructions:

1. Mix all oils.
2. Add vitamin E and essential oils.
3. Let cool slightly before pouring.
4. Pour into 50 ml glass roll-on bottles
5. Place Thai chili or cayenne in each bottle.
6. Label.

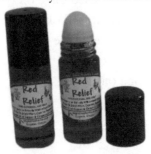

Sore Stop

Remedy for cold sores. Works.

Ingredients:

- 2 cups calendula infused olive oil
- 2 cups St. John's wort infused olive oil
- 2 cups lemon balm infused olive oil
- 1/8 oz cajeput essential oil
- 1/8 oz camphor essential oil
- 6 oz beeswax
- 1 tbsp vitamin E

Instructions:

1. Melt wax in a double boiler.
2. Add to oils and heat over low heat until well mixed.
3. Remove from heat, add vitamin E and essential oils.
4. Let cool slightly before pouring.
5. Pour into ½ oz glass jars.
6. Label.

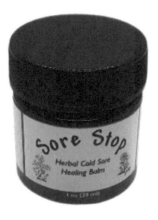

Trauma Oil
Our arnica remedy for bruising, not for open wounds.

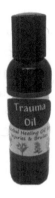

Ingredients:
- 3 cups arnica infused olive oil
- 1 cup comfrey infused olive oil
- 1 cup St. John's wort infused olive oil
- 1 cup calendula infused olive oil
- 1 tbsp vitamin E

Instructions:
1. Mix all oils.
2. Add vitamin E
3. Pour into 2 oz green plastic bottles with flip tops.
4. Label.

Smoking Blends

Full Bloom Smoking Blend
Roses add a nice touch.

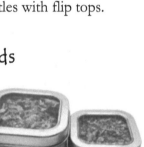

Ingredients:
- 3 cups dried mullein
- 1 cup dried catnip
- 1 cup dried damiana
- ½ cup dried lavender
- ½ cup dried rose petals

Instructions:
1. Mix all herbs well.
2. Pour into 2 and 4 oz window tins.
3. Label.

Soul Soother Smoking Blend
Light and mellow.

Ingredients:

- 3 cups dried mullein
- 1 cup dried mugwort
- 1 cup dried damiana
- 1 cup dried chamomile
- ½ cup dried lavender

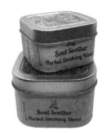

Instructions:

4. Mix all herbs well.
5. Pour into 2 and 4 oz window tins.
6. Label.

Syrups & Elixirs—Medicinal

Herbal Cough Syrup
Some of my products I am going to keep making even after retiring because they are just so good. This is one of them.

Ingredients:

- 1 ½ gallons distilled water
- 1 lb organic cane sugar
- 2 oz wild cherry bark
- 4 oz coltsfoot
- 4 oz mullein
- 2 oz slippery elm
- 2 oz osha root
- 4 oz marshmallow
- 1 oz ginger powder

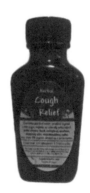

Instructions:

1. Boil decoction of cherry bark and osha root for 1 hr.
2. Turn off heat, add the rest of herbs to the pot, cover and let sit for ½ hour.
3. Strain.
4. Add the sugar to the hot tea and stir while the sugar dissolves and slowly boil until thickens.
5. Remove from heat.
6. Pour into 3 oz glass bottles.
7. Label.

Elder Ally Syrups

Another one of my "brilliant ideas" that fell flat. I take a lot of tinctures and they often taste terrible. I thought if they were more palatable, I would take them more often. These are tincture and syrup combinations specifically designed for older people. Did a lot of research to find the right formulas. Did not catch on. If someone is looking for a unique product, this is it. I would love to see these live on.

Brain Booster

Besides memory herbs included, blueberries cross the blood-brain barrier and are good for memory.

Ingredients:

- 16 cups sugar
- 8 cups of filtered water
- 4 cups dried blueberry powder
- 2 cups gotu kola tincture
- 2 cups ginkgo tincture
- 2 cups sage tincture
- 1 cup brahmi tincture

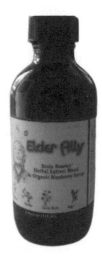

Instructions:
1. Boil water.
2. Add sugar and blueberry powder until dissolved.
3. Remove from heat, when cool add tinctures.
4. Pour into 2 & 4 oz glass dropper bottles.
5. Label.

Heart Strong

Hawthorn berry syrup makes a nice base for the other herbs.

Ingredients:
- 16 cups sugar
- 8 cups of filtered water
- 4 cups hawthorn berry powder
- 2 cups hibiscus tincture
- 2 cups motherwort tincture
- 2 cups white willow tincture
- 1 cup red clover tincture

Instructions:
1. Boil water.
2. Add sugar and hawthorn berry powder until dissolved.
3. Remove from heat, when cool add tinctures.
4. Pour into 2 & 4 oz glass dropper bottles.
5. Label.

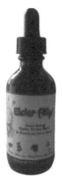

Move Well—Arthritis Blend

Wish I had more of this made. If anyone makes it, please send me some.

Ingredients:

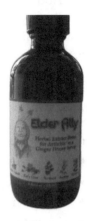

- 4 cups honey.
- 4 cups filtered water
- 1 cup cat's claw tincture
- 1 cup ginger tincture
- ½ cup black cohosh tincture
- ½ cup devil's club tincture
- ½ cup feverfew tincture
- ½ cup burdock

Instructions:

1. Heat water until honey is dissolved.
2. Remove from heat, when cool add tinctures.
3. Pour into 2 & 4 oz glass dropper bottles.
4. Label.

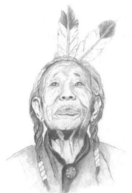

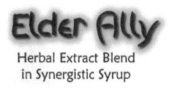

Elder Ally

Herbal Extract Blend
in Synergistic Syrup

Age Active - Age Well - Age Strong

Elderberry Syrup

We made it for 30 years until you could buy it anywhere cheaper than the cost of honey and bottles.

Ingredients:
- 1 gallon filtered water
- 1 gallon fresh elderberry, or use half dried elderberry
- 8 cups honey

Instructions:
1. Be sure to remove stems from fresh elderberries.
2. Boil elderberries in water on low heat for 30 minutes.
3. Strain.
4. Heat back up a little, add honey and mix well.
5. Remove from heat.
6. Pour into 2 oz glass bottles.
7. Label.

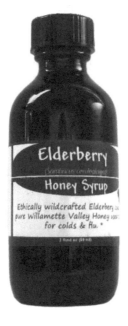

Lemon Ginger Elixer

One of the first products in the early days of OCF we made especially for dry scratchy throats because the dust was a real problem. Also good for tummy upsets.

Ingredients:
- 8 cups honey
- 1/2 qt dried ginger root
- 2 cups fresh ginger root
- 1/2 qt ginger honey
- 2 cups dried rosehips
- juice of 1 lemon
- 1 cup lemon tincture
- 2 cups ginger tincture
- ½ cup rosehip tincture

Instructions:
1. Boil decoction of ginger root for 1 hr.
2. Turn off heat, add rosehips, cover and let sit for ½ hour.
3. Strain.
4. Add the honey to the hot tea until dissolved.
5. Remove from heat.
6. Add lemon juice.
7. Add tinctures.
8. Pour into 2 and 4 oz glass bottles.
9. Label.

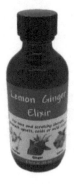

Revive Herbal Elixir

It is sorta like an organic chocolate "Red Bull" except you add it to another drink, or take a tablespoon or two. The entire crew depended on it for tear down and pack up when the festivals were over.

Ingredients:
- 13 quarts filtered water.
- 2 cups guayusa leaf
- 2 cups green tea
- 1 cup yerba mate
- 1 cup ground green coffee beans
- 16 cups sugar
- 1½ cups cocoa powder
- 1/8 cup green coffee tincture
- 4 tbsp yohimbe tincture
- 4 tbsp guayusa tincture

Instructions:
1. Boil water and turn off heat, make an infusion with tea and coffee let steep for ½ hour.
2. Strain.
3. Slowly heat the tea up, add sugar until it dissolves.
4. Add cocoa powder.
5. Remove from heat.
6. Add tinctures. Mix well.
7. Pour into 2 and 4 oz glass bottles.
8. Label.

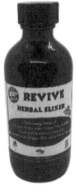

Teas

Immuni-tea
This tea has long proven its worth.

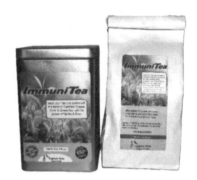

Ingredients:
- 6 cups elderberry flowers
- 4 cups green tea
- 4 cups dried nettle leaf
- 2 cup dried elderberries
- 2 cup white tea

Instructions:
1. Mix all herbs well.
2. Weigh 2 oz in each bag and 4 oz in tins.
3. Label.

Sereni-tea
Calming and soothing.

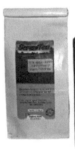 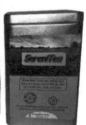

Ingredients:
- 6 cups lemon balm
- 4 cups chamomile
- 2 cups passionflower
- 2 cup lavender

Instructions:
1. Mix all herbs well.
2. Weigh 2 oz in each bag and 4 oz in tins.
3. Label.

Wild Hipster
Read the back label on this. It is hilarious, Trillium's work again.

Ingredients:
- 6 cups lemon balm
- 6 cups spearmint
- 4 cups raspberry leaf
- 4 cups rosehips

Instructions:
1. Mix all herbs well.
2. Weigh 2 oz in each bag and 4 oz in tins.
3. Label.

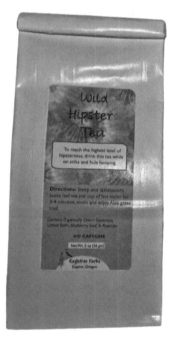

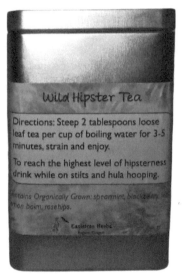

Wild Hipster Tea

Directions: Steep 2 tablespoons loose leaf tea per cup of boiling water for 3-5 minutes, strain and enjoy.

To reach the highest level of hipsterness drink while on stilts and hula hooping.

Contains Organically Grown: spearmint, blackberry leaf, lemon balm, rosehips.

Eagletree Herbs
Eugene, Oregon

Eagletree Tinctures

Alcohol Tincture Blends

I keep formulas simple and do extensive research for each one. Use these or make your own. Just pay attention to new research. I have had to change formulas over the years.

Allergy Relief: butterbur, nettles, angelica, feverfew.

Arthritis Formula: cat's claw, burdock, nettles, black cohosh, feverfew.

Brain Boost: brahmi, gotu kola, ginkgo, sage, blessed thistle.

Calm: lemon balm, passionflower.

Cold & Flu: elderberry, yarrow, echinacea, lomatium, sage.

Crone Care: black cohosh, vitex, licorice, blue cohosh.

Digestive Bitters: angelica root, fennel leaf, burdock root, yarrow leaves and flower.

Heart Health: red clover, artichoke, hibiscus, immune boost, astragalus, cat's claw, echinacea, nettles, white tea.

Libido Rising: horny goat weed, muira puama, damiana, yohimbe, ginseng.

Male Tonic: saw palmetto, pygeum, nettles, pipsissewa, ginseng.

Nursing Mother: fenugreek, blessed thistle, alfalfa, borage, fennel.

Pain Relief: skullcap, cramp bark, white willow, California poppy, Jamaican dogwood.

Sleep Well: valerian root, chamomile flowers, skullcap leaf.

2:30 Tooth Tincture: comfrey, yarrow, red root, clove essential oil.

UTI Formula: urva ursi, usnea, pau d'arco, couch grass, cleavers.

Yeast Away: pau d'arco bark, spilanthes, oregano, usnea.

Not alcohol - infused oil. **Ear Oil:** olive oil, garlic, mullein, vitamin E.

Single Tinctures

Giving up making these is like giving up one of my children, each offers unique properties. I spent hours looking for the perfect picture of the herbs to put on the label even though they were so small they could hardly be seen.

- Alfalfa: *Medicago sativa*
- Angelica Rt: *Angelica archangelica*
- Ashwagandha: *Withania somnifera*
- Astragalus: *Astragalus membranaceus*
- Black Cohosh: *Actaea racemosa* (previously *Cimicifuga racemosa*)
- Black Walnut: *Juglans nigra*
- Blessed Thistle: *Cnicus benedictus*

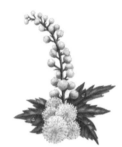

Black Cohosh

- Black Cohosh: *Actaea racemosa* (previously *Cimicifuga racemosa*)
- Blue Cohosh: *Caulophyllum thalictroides*
- Brahmi: *Bacopa monnieri*
- Burdock: *Arctium lappa*
- Butterbur: *Petasites hybridus*
- California Poppy: *Eschscholzia californica*
- Cascara Sagrada: *Rhamnus purshiana*
- Cat's Claw: *Uncaria tomentosa*
- Chamomile: *Matricaria chamomilla*
- Chasteberry: *Vitex agnus-castus*
- Cleavers: *Galium aparine*
- Comfrey: *Symphytum officinale*
- Cornsilk: *Zea mays*
- Cramp Bark: *Viburnum opulus*
- Dandelion Root: *Taraxacum officinale*
- Devil's Club: *Oplopanax horridus*

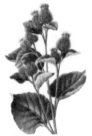

Burdock

- Echinacea: *Echinacea purpurea & Echinacea angustifolia*
- Elecampane: *Inula helenium*
- Elderberry: *Sambucus nigra*
- Fennel: *Foeniculum vulgare*
- Fenugreek: *Trigonella foenum-graecum*
- Feverfew: *Tanacetum parthenium*
- Ginko: *Ginkgo biloba*
- Gotu Kola: *Centella asiatica*
- Goat's Rue: *Galega officinalis*
- Gymnema: *Gymnema sylvestre*
- Horsetail: *Equisetum arvense*
- Hops: *Humulus lupulus*
- Kava Kava: *Piper methysticum*
- Lemon Balm: *Melissa officinalis*
- Licorice Root: *Glycyrrhiza glabra*
- Lomatium: *Lomatium dissectum*
- Lungwort: *Pulmonaria officinalis*
- Marshmallow root: *Althaea officinalis*
- Milk Thistle: *Silybum marianum*
- Milky Oat: *Avena sativa*
- Motherwort: *Leonurus cardiaca*
- Nettles: *Urtica dioica*
- Oregon Grape: *Mahonia aquifolium*
- Osha Root: *Ligusticum porteri*
- Passionflower: *Passiflora incarnata*
- Pau d'arco: *Tabebuia impetiginosa*
- Pipsissewa: *Chimaphila umbellata*
- Red Clover: *Trifolium pratense*
- Red Root: *Ceanothus americanus*
- Red Raspberry: *Rubus idaeus*
- Reishi Mushroom: *Ganoderma lucidum*
- Sage: *Salvia officinalis*
- Saw Palmetto: *Serenoa repens*

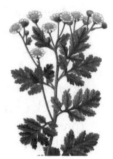

Feverfew

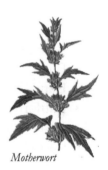

Motherwort

- Shepherd's Purse: *Capsella bursa-pastoris*
- St John's Wort: *Hypericum perforatum*
- Skullcap: *Scutellaria lateriflora*
- Usnea: *Usnea spp.*
- Valerian Root: *Valeriana officinalis*
- White Willow Bark: *Salix alba*
- Yarrow: *Achillea millefolium*
- Yellow Dock Root: *Rumex crispus*

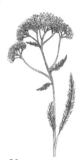

Glycerin Tinctures:

Yarrow

- Ashwagandha: *Withania somnifera*
- Chamomile: *Matricaria chamomilla*
- Elderberry: *Sambucus nigra*
- Fennel: *Foeniculum vulgare*
- Lemon Balm: *Melissa officinalis*
- Licorice: *Glycyrrhiza glabra*
- Milk Thistle: *Silybum marianum*
- Spearmint: *Mentha spicata*

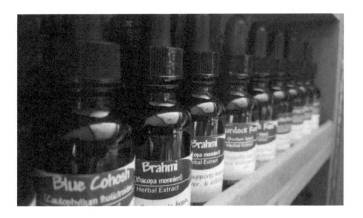

Kratom

I make kratom tinctures for those who want the occasional convenience, but the tea is much better. Kratom is a subject of considerable controversy, some calling it an herb, others a drug. When brewed into tea, this plant medicine, utilized for millennia by indigenous peoples of Southeast Asia, 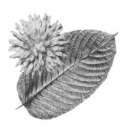 offers potent therapeutic benefits. Conversely, when ingested as a pill, concentrate, or extract, it veers into drug-like territory.

Personally, kratom has significantly aided me, particularly in managing chronic pain stemming from my car accident.

Belonging to the coffee family, it can be as habit-forming as caffeine. Due to its euphoric effects, kratom is also sought after as a legal recreational "high," available for purchase online and in head/smoke shops. This emphasis on its recreational use undermines its medicinal value. While currently legal in most U.S. states, it remains under scrutiny by the DEA. Given its efficacy in combating prescription drug dependence, suspicions have arisen about potential lobbying efforts by pharmaceutical companies to criminalize this natural remedy.

Research indicates that kratom acts as an analgesic, euphoric, antidepressant, anti-anxiety agent, and immune booster. It has also shown promise in reducing blood pressure, combating viruses, managing diabetes, and suppressing appetite. Certain alkaloids in kratom function as μ-opioid receptor antagonists, akin to pharmaceutical pain relievers. Despite this similarity, kratom is not derived from the opium poppy. Some individuals use it for enhanced mental clarity and productivity, as an alternative to ADHD medications like Adderall. In Southeast Asia, its traditional uses span stimulant effects, antidiarrheal properties, cough suppression, enhancement of sexual stamina, treatment of intestinal parasites, and application as a wound poultice. It is even incorporated into a popular energy drink. Studies have highlighted its efficacy in aiding withdrawal from prescription painkillers, opioids, methadone, and methamphetamine (Greenmeier 2013).

For individuals with chronic pain conditions, kratom not only alleviates pain but also provides an energy boost that facilitates greater physical activity, thereby promoting overall health.

Safety Considerations: At normal doses, kratom is generally deemed safe, supported by its extensive historical usage and scientific investigations. Approximately 70% of adult males in Southern Thailand consume kratom daily without significant adverse effects. However, sourcing kratom from reputable suppliers and using whole leaves, tea, or pure powder is crucial. Extracts and capsules may contain impurities or additives. Processing to extract specific alkaloids can transform a safe herbal remedy into a potentially hazardous substance. Consequently, kratom should be approached with caution and respect. While overdoses may cause nausea and vomiting, there are no documented fatalities from the ingestion of pure leaf or powder as a tea.

Kratom should be avoided during pregnancy and nursing. Limited research exists on potential drug interactions, prompting individuals taking prescription medications to be careful combining kratom with other drugs.

While smaller daily doses of pure leaf are safe, tolerance may necessitate increased dosages over time to maintain effectiveness. Therefore, many kratom advocates recommend restricting usage to a few times per week. Users who consume larger daily doses may experience mild withdrawal symptoms upon cessation, similar to those associated with coffee.

Acknowledgements

A special acknowledgement to Sue Sierralupe, an incredible herbalist who worked for Eagletree Herbs part time, for a brief time, a long time ago. Part of her job was to enter all the recipes we had written into the computer. She told me she thought I should publish the recipes, but I demurred, thinking someday I might sell the business and the recipes were my hard-earned intellectual property. But with her work and inspiration, it was easier to get this book out, as most of the recipes were on the computer.

There are too many people that helped over the years to list all the names, but much gratitude to Janet and Jerry Russell, who continue to believe support me and the work I do.

I want to extend a special thank you to my home helpers. Since my car accident, everyday tasks have become difficult and time-consuming. Their assistance allows me to write. They are my friends and support system, always there when needed. Thank you, Shari Arthur, Sharon Cohen, and Cindy Herzog.

Thank you to editor Lili Marlene Booth and my publishing assistant, Mary Glor Cuda, for being so much help.

And of course all the interns who have helped make medicines over the decades, wish I remembered all your names.

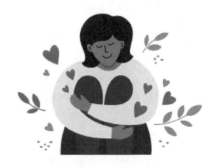

About the Author

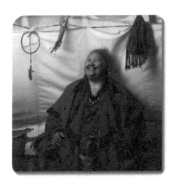

Daphne Singingtree is an educator in plant medicine, midwifery, and emergency preparedness, a water protector and land defender. While she is best known for her works in midwifery, such as the _Birthsong Midwifery Workbook_, the Emergency Guide to Obstetric Complications, and Training Midwives: A Guide for Preceptors, she recently debuted her first novel, Circle of the Earth, A Time Travel Saga for a Sustainable Future.

Daphne started midwifery in 1974, leading to an active practice in home and birth center settings until her retirement in 2002. Her influence extends beyond her practice, as she played a pivotal role in shaping midwifery education and accreditation. She was the founder and director of the Birthsong School of Midwifery from 1979 to 1989 and the Oregon School of Midwifery from 1993 to 2002. Daphne holds a Masters in Education with a concentration on learning with technology.

Daphne is also an urban homesteader, promoting permaculture, emergency preparation, and food resilience. She emphasizes the importance of emergency preparedness, not just for personal survival but also for the ability to aid others.

She has remained dedicated to learning and teaching about plant medicine throughout her life, a passion she continues to pursue.

Her heritage includes Lakota from the Standing Rock Tribe, Spanish, and Scottish. She is the mother of four grown children and the grandmother of eight. She calls Eugene, Oregon, home.

Feedback is Appreciated

This first edition of the book has much room for improvement, your comments, even criticism, will make the next edition better. Contact me at <u>daphnesingingtree@gmail.com</u>

Reviews on Amazon and other book outlets really help. You can order this book directly from my website at eagletreepress.com either paperback or ebook.

Other Books by Daphne Singingtree

Available at eagletreepress.com, Amazon and other <u>outlets.</u>

Midwifery

Birthsong Midwifery Workbook
Basic Level Coloring Book and Study Guide.
Training Midwives A Guide for Preceptors
Emergency Guide to Obstetric Complications

Fiction

Circle for the Earth A Time Travel Saga for a Sustainable Future

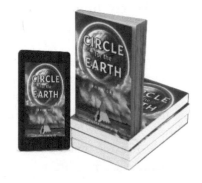

The Earth grants humanity an extraordinary second chance. Imagine hurtling a South Dakota Indian casino and its surroundings thirty miles back in time to 1791, before the Louisiana Purchase. This gripping novel explores a collision of eras—a modern world mingling with the past—unraveling a narrative ripe with survival, cultural clashes, and deep human connections.

Glossary of Herbal Preparation

Capsule: Dried powdered herb, contained in a gelatin capsule (pill covering). Capsules come in various sizes, denoted by the number of zeroes, for example, 000 capsules.

Cold Compress: An absorbent folded cloth, dipped in a cold fluid (cold water or a cold herbal infusion) and applied topically to a body area.

Cordial: Cordials are herbs (often fresh herbs or fruit juices) mixed with alcohol, such as brandy and left to macerate. After strained, an equal amount of sweetener is added.

Cream: A mixture of water and fat or oil applied to the skin.

Decant: To strain an infusion or tincture, saving the fluid portion and discarding the plant matter.

Decoction: Water-based preparation of bark, roots, leaves, flowers, berries, or seeds simmered in boiling water.

Electuary: Medicine mixed with honey or another sweet substance

Elixir: A syrup with alcohol as a preservative.

Essential Oil: Distillation of volatile oils derived from aromatic plants. These are *extremely potent and must be diluted* in a carrier oil or fluid in the proper dilution before use.

Extract: A tincture of a plant, usually made with a standardized ratio.

Fixed Oil: A nonvolatile oil (plant constituent) produced by hot or cold infusion (preparation).

Fomentation: The localized application of alternating hot and cold compresses to increase circulation and relieve pain and swelling.

Galenical: A medicine in a standard formula prepared from plants.

Hot Compress: An absorbent folded cloth, dipped in hot fluid (for example, hot water or an herbal infusion) applied topically to an area.

Infused oils: An oil-based preparation in which the plant matter is packed in a jar with vegetable oil (often olive oil) to draw out its properties.

Infusion: Water-based preparation in which flowers, leaves, or stems are brewed like tea.

Inhalation: Breathing of medicinally infused steam or liquid through the nasal passages.

Liniment: External medication applied by rubbing.

Maceration: Maceration is the process of soaking the herb or plant matter in the menstruum, or solvent, to soak up an herb's constituents.

Marc: Marc is what's left over after maceration and extraction into a menstruum.

Menstruum: Solvent used to extract compounds from herbs, like alcohol, glycerin, or vinegar.

Ointment: A blend of fats or oils that form a protective layer over the skin.

Oxymel: A combination of vinegar and honey.

Poultice: A moist, soft mass or paste made of herbs or other substances usually applied hot to affected area to alleviate pain and reduce swelling.

Simple: An herb used on its own.

Steam Inhalation: 5-10 drops of essential oil added to one liter of very hot water or a hot infusion of an herb placed in a container. The container is then covered with a towel, into which the person sticks their head to breathe the herbal steam.

Suppositories: An herbal combination (cocoa butter or powdered herb mixed with an essential oil or infused oil) shaped into long, thin cylinders and frozen to harden them. They are then used by inserting them into the rectum or vagina.

Syrup: An infusion or decoction combined with honey or sugar as a preservative. Helpful for sore throats, coughs, children's remedies, and to enhance the palatability of unpleasantly flavored herbs.

Tincture: Plant medicine prepared by soaking and straining herbs in alcohol, vinegar, or glycerin.

Topical: An herbal remedy to be applied to the body surface.

Volatile Oil: Plant constituent distilled to produce essential oil.

Glossary of Medicinal Actions of Herbs

Abortifacient: Causes miscarriage.

Adaptogenic: Helps the body adapt to stress and supports normal function.

Alternative: promotes a gradual and beneficial change in the body.

Anabolic: Promotes tissue growth.

Analgesic: Reduces pain.

Anaphrodisiac: Inhibits libido and sexual activity.

Anesthetic: Numbs perception of external sensations.

Anodyne: Relieves pain.

Anthelmintic: Expels or destroys parasitic worms.

Anthraquinones: Irritate the intestinal wall causing bowel movement.

Anti-asthmatic: Relieves the symptoms of asthma.

Anti-biliousness: Relieves biliousness.

Antibiotic: Destroys or inhibits micro-organisms.

Anticoagulant: Prevents blood clotting.

Antidiarrheal: Combats and arrests diarrhea.

Antiemetic: Stops vomiting.

Antifungal: Combats fungal infections.

Anti-galactagogue: Diminishes milk production.

Anti-inflammatory: Reduces inflammation.

Antilytic: Prevents formation of urinary calculi.

Antimicrobial: Destroys or inhibits micro-organisms.

Antioxidant: Prevents oxidation and breakdown of tissues.

Antipyretic: Reduces fever.

Antirheumatic: Relieves rheumatism.

Antiscorbutic: Cures or prevents scurvy.

Antiseptic: Destroys or inhibits micro-organisms that cause infection.

Antispasmodic: Relieves muscle spasms or reduces muscle tone.

Antitussive: Soothes and relieves coughing.

Aperient: Mild laxative.

Aperitive: Stimulates the appetite.

Aphrodisiac: Excites libido and sexual activity.

Aromatic: Spicy stimulant.

Astringent: Tightens mucous membranes and skin, reducing secretions and bleeding.

Bitter: Stimulates secretions of saliva and digestive juices, increasing appetite.

Bowel Irritant: Increases peristalsis of the gastrointestinal tract, causing diarrhea.

Carcinogenic: Causes cancer.

Cardiotonic: Improves heart function.

Carminative: Relieves digestive gas and indigestion.

Cathartic: Powerful purgative (strong laxative).

Cholagogue: Stimulates the release of bile from the gallbladder.

Circulatory Stimulant: Increases blood flow, usually to a given area, e.g., hands and feet.

Demulcent: Coats, soothes, and protects body surfaces such as the gastric mucous membranes.

Depurative: Detoxifying agent.

Detoxification: Aids in the removal of toxins and waste products from the body.

Diaphoretic: Induces sweating.

Diuretic: Stimulates urine flow.

Emetic: Causes vomiting.

Emmenagogue: Promotes menstruation.

Emollient: Softens or soothes the skin.

Esculent: Eatable as food.

Estrogenic: With a similar action to estrogen.

Expectorant: Stimulates coughing and helps clear phlegm.

Febrifuge: Abates or reduces fever.

Fetotoxic: Potentially harmful to the growing fetus.

Galactagogue: Increases milk production.
Genotoxic: Prevents normal growth.

Hallucinogenic: Causes visions or hallucinations.
Hemolytic: Destroys red blood cells.
Hemostatic: Stops or reduces bleeding.
Hepatic: Affects the liver.
Hepatotoxic: Damaging to the liver.
Herpetic: Remedies for eruptions of the skin.
Hormonal: Contains precursors to or alters the body's
    production of hormones.
Hypnotic: Induces sleep.
Hypoglycemic: Reduces the blood sugar level.

Immune Stimulant: Stimulates the immune system to
    defend the body from infection.

Laxative: Promotes evacuation of the bowels.
Lithotriptic: Helps dissolve kidney stones.

Maturating: Ripens or brings boils and ulcers to a head.
Mucilaginous: Gelatinous, viscous substance soothing to
    inflamed parts.
Mutagen: Interferes with normal cell growth.
Mydriatic: Dilates the pupil of the eye.

Narcotic: Causes drowsiness or stupor and relieves pain.
Nauseant: Produces nausea and/or vomiting.
Nervine: Restores the nerves; relaxes the nervous system.
Nutritive: Providing nutritional value.

Oxytocic: Induces contractions of the uterus, speeds
    labor.

Parasiticide: Kills parasites.
Pectoral: Acts on the lungs.
Purgative: Promotes rapid and extreme bowel evacuation.

Pyrrolizidine alkaloids: Potentially toxic alkaline compounds.

Refrigerant: Having a cooling quality.
Rubefacient: Stimulates blood flow, produces skin reddening.

Sedative: Reduces activity and nervous excitement.
Sialagogue: Stimulates the flow of saliva to aid digestion.
Spasmolytic: Relaxes muscles.
Stimulant: Increases the rate of activity and nervous excitement.
Stomachic: A gastric stimulant.
Styptic: Stops bleeding when applied topically.
Sudorific: Produces profuse perspiration.

Teratogenic: Interferes with the normal development of fetus.
Tonic: Invigorating or strengthening.

Uterine Relaxant: Diminishes spasms of the uterine muscle, interferes with effective labor.
Uterine Stimulant: Causes the uterus to contract.

Vasoconstrictor: Contacts and narrows blood vessels.
Vasodilator: Relaxes and widens blood vessels.
Vermifuge: Expe ls intestinal worms.

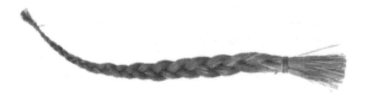

Sweet Grass (Hierochloe odorata)

Medicinal Actions Word Search

```
            P G H
          A A E N V S Z
        O S E C J U X C M
      S E U S T O G B D E X
    E U G O G O T C A L A G C
  N X Q L N R R N N E R V I N E
  X P B R I T A E W U W A B C S
T D E W L G N L I M G E M E T I C
Y T I C C Y A E A L F O V R H E E P W
Y N U T I K L I S L O G I Z B B A P Y
G D R O T E I C T O C A T H A R T I C
X K E R E U C A R M I N A T I V E I F
  U T A P T U F I E T E G W W D T O
    I N R T M E N G E M R R L A M
    C T E I A B G U R M U T P V U
      S H C X U E F O E P E N H
          L R N I H U H
            U T R P Q
            X M B A W
              N E I
              R F D
```

1. Tightens mucous membranes and skin, reducing secretions & bleeding
2. Relieves digestive gas and indigestion
3. Powerful purgative (strong laxative)
4. Coats, soothes, and protects gastric mucous membranes
6. Stimulates urine flow
7. Causes vomiting
8. Promotes menstruation
9. Softens or soothes the skin
10. Stimulates coughing and helps clear phlegm from the throat and chest
11. Abates or reduces fever
12. Increases milk
13. Affects the liver
14. Remedies for eruptions of the skin
15. Gelatinous, viscous substance that is soothing to inflamed parts
16. Restores the nerves; relaxes the nervous system
17. Acts on the lungs
18. Promotes rapid and extreme bowel movements
19. Stimulates blood flow, produces reddening of the skin

From the Birthsong Midwifery Workbook 6ᵗʰ edition by Daphne Singingtree

Bulk Herb Directory

List from Plant Savers United for companies who offer bulk herbs that are organically cultivated or wildcrafted in an environmentally responsible manner that ensures adequate regeneration of wild plant colonies.

Bees' Dance Medicinal Herb Farm
1174 Will Grimes Rd, Hyde Park, VT 05655 Phone: 802-888-8589
A bio-dynamic and certified organic farm offering over 50 varieties of medicinal herbs sold dried or fresh by the pound.

Bighorn Botanicals, Inc.
PO Box 133, Noxon, MT 59853 Phone: 406-847-5597
www.bighornbotanicals.com
 Bulk wholesale and retail of sustainably wildcrafted or grown without chemicals medicinal herbs native and naturalized to western Montana.

Blessed Herbs
109 Barre Plains Rd, Oakham, MA 01068 Phone: 508-882-3839
www.blessedherbs.com
Offers over 600 premium quality bulk herbs and herbal products. All of our herbs and herbal products are free of any fumigation, irradiation or synthetic chemicals. We offer certified organic herbs whenever possible.

Cate Farm
135 Cate Farm Road, Plainfield, VT 05667 Phone: 802-454-7157
www.catefarm.com
Certified organically grown echinacea purpurea roots and flowers, burdock root, dandelion root and valerian root.

Flack Family Farm
3971 Pumpkin Village Road, Enosburg Falls, VT 05450
Phone: 802-933-7752 www.flackfamilyfarm.com
Certified organic farm practicing biodynamic methods. Black cohosh, Solomon's seal, blue cohosh and St. John's wort flowers available.

Frontier Natural Products Co-op
P.O. Box 299, Norway, IA 52318 Phone: 800-669-3275
www.frontiercoop.com
Supplies hundreds of medicinal and culinary herbs including many
certified organic which include at risk plants such as goldenseal,
American ginseng, black cohosh, slippery elm and wild yam.

Healing Spirits Herb Farm & Education Center
9198 State Route 415 Avoca, NY 14809 Phone: 607-566-2701
www.healingspiritsherbfarm.com
Over 60 species of certified organic medicinal herbs available.

Loess Roots
PO Box 877, Stanton, NE 68779 Phone: 402-439-5256
Email: rodangerorth@yahoo.com
Can provide small quantities of quality fresh mature roots of
American ginseng (very large roots, 12= years), goldenseal,
bloodroot and black cohosh for tinctures, salves or drying.

MoonBranch Botanicals
5294 Yellow Creek Road, Robbinsville, NC 28771
Phone: 828-479-2788 www.moonbranch.com
Sustainably and ethically produced herbs native to Southeastern
North Carolina, including many at risk species.

Mountain Gardens
546 Shuford Creek Road, Burnsville, NC 28714
Phone: 828-675-5664 www.mountaingardensherbs.com
Offer almost all of the Eastern U.S. at risk herbs. Specializing in
seeds of native and oriental medicinal herbs.

Mountain Rose Herbs
P.O. Box 50220, Eugene, OR 97405
Phone: 800-879-3337
www.mountainroseherbs.com
The majority of herbs are certified organically grown.

Owl Mountain Herbs

75 Owl Mountain Road, Clyde, NC 28721 Phone: 828-627-2769
Grower of naturally cultivated herbs (not certified organic)
including black cohosh, blue cohosh, goldenseal, ginseng and wild
yam.

Pacific Botanicals

4840 Fish Hatchery Road, Grants Pass, OR 97527
Phone: 541-479-7777 www.pacificbotanicals.com
200 certified organic herbs and spices including medicinal, culinary,
seaweed and green food.

Sonoma County Herb Exchange

PO Box 2162, Sebastopol, CA 95472 Phone: 707-824-1447
www.sonomaherbs.com
A network of dedicated herb growers from Sonoma County and
adjoining regions of Northern California; all follow organic or
biodynamic methods.

Spring Mountain Herbs of Vermont

4570 Ireland Road, Starksboro, VT 05487 Phone: 413-320-1920
Email: margigregory@comcast.net Western, Chinese and Ayurvedic
tonic and medicinal herbs available, organic/biodynamically grown
(but not certified) or responsibly wildcrafted.

Starwest Botanicals

11253 Trade Center Drive, Rancho Cordova, CA 95742
Phone: 800-800-4372 www.starwest-botanicals.com
Offer a wide selection of botanicals, herbs & spices - over 550
varieties, including many certified organic culinary, medicinal and
Chinese herbs. Certified organic processor and Kosher certified
facility.

Zack Woods Herb Farm 278 Mead Road, Hyde Park, VT 05655
Phone: 802-888-7278 www.zackwoodsherbs.com
Offer over 40 species of dried or freshly harvested herbs including
arnica, black cohosh, bloodroot, Echinacea, goldenseal, lobelia and
pleurisy root. NOFA certified organic.

Herbal Organizations & Publications

from *Chestnut School of Herbal Medicine*

American Botanical Council
Publishes the quarterly Herbal Gram, which focuses on medical herbalism and the herbal industry. Website has many searchable databases related to scientific research on medicinal herbs.

American Herbalists Guild
The AHG is an association of herbal practitioners. Annual conference held in changing locations. Membership includes many educational benefits.

Herbal Roots Zine
An herbal e-magazine for children! Planting a seed of knowledge for a lifetime of herbal wisdom.

Medical Herbalism
Medical Herbalism is a journal for clinical herbal practitioners. Free e-journal issues are available via this link.

Plant Healer Magazine
Plant Healer is the paperless quarterly e-journal of the new folk herbalism movement – it's a downloadable, beautifully illustrated, full color PDF publication. An annual condensed print version is also available.

United Plant Savers
A stalwart organization devoted to protecting the native medicinal plants of the United States and Canada and their native habitat while ensuring an abundant renewable supply of medicinal plants for generations to come.

Bibliography & References

Adkins, J. E., Boyer, E. W., & McCurdy, C. R. (2011). Mitragyna speciosa, a psychoactive tree from Southeast Asia with opioid activity. *Current Topics in Medicinal Chemistry, 11*, 1165–1175.

Ahmed, M., Hwang, J. H., Choi, S., & Han, D. (2017). Safety classification of herbal medicines used among pregnant women in Asian countries: A systematic review. *BMC Complementary and Alternative Medicine, 17*. https://doi.org/10.1186/s12906-017-1995-6

Batume, C., Mulongo, I. M., Ludlow, R., et al. (2024). Evaluating repellence properties of catnip essential oil against the mosquito species *Aedes aegypti* using a Y-tube olfactometer. *Scientific Reports, 14*, 2269. https://doi.org/10.1038/s41598-024-52715-y

Beckett, A. H., Shellard, E. J., Phillipson, J. D., & Lee, C. M. (1966). The *Mitragyna* species of Asia. Part VII. Indole alkaloids from the leaves of *Mitragyna speciosa* Korth. *Planta Medica, 14*, 277–288.

Botpiboon, O., Prutipanlai, S., Janchawee, B., & Thainchaiwattana, S. (2009). Effect of caffeine and codeine on antinociceptive activity of alkaloid extract from leaves of kratom (*Mitragyna speciosa* Korth.). Paper presented at The 35th Congress on Science and Technology of Thailand. Retrieved from http://www.scientificamerican.com/article.cfm?id=should-kratom-be-legal

Cech, R. (2016). *Making Plant Medicine*. Herbal Reads LLC.

Croom, E. M. 1983. Documenting and evaluating herbal remedies. Econ. Bot. 37: 13-27.

Culpeper, N. 1653. The English physician enlarged. George Sawbridge. London, England. Elvin-Lewis, M. (2001). Should we be concerned about herbal remedies. *Journal of Ethnopharmacology, 75*(2-3), 141–164. https://doi.org/10.1016/S0378-8741(00)00394-9

Field, E. (1921). Mitragynine and mitraversine, two new alkaloids from species of *Mitragyne. Journal of the Chemical Society. Transactions, 119*, 887–891.

Francis Brinker, N.D. (1997). *Herb Contraindications and Drug Interactions*. Eclectic Institute.

GholamiF, NeisaniSamaniL, KashanianM, NaseriM, Hosseini AF, Hashemi NejadSA. (2016). Onset of Labor in Post-Term Pregnancy by Chamomile. *Iran Red Crescent Med J, 18*(11), e19871. https://doi.org/10.5812/ircmj.19871

Gladstar, R. (1993). *Herbal Healing for Women*. Simon and Schuster.

Green, J. (2000). *The Herbal Medicine-Maker's Handbook: A Home Manual*. Crossing Press.

Grieve, M. (1931). *A modern herbal; the medicinal, culinary, cosmetic and economic properties, cultivation and folk-lore of herbs, grasses, fungi, shrubs, & trees with all their modern scientific uses*. New York: Harcourt, Brace & Company.

Greenemeier, L. (2013, September 30). Should kratom use be legal. Retrieved from http://www.scientificamerican.com/article.cfm?id=should-kratom-be-legal

Gold, J. & W. Gates. 1980. Herbal abortifacients. J. American Med. Assoc. 243: 1365, 1366.

Hoffmann, D. 1993. An elder's herbal: natural techniques for promoting health & vitality. Healing Arts Press. Rochester, VT. 266 pp.

Hoffmann, D. (editor). 1994. The information sourcebook of herbal medicine. Crossing Press. Freedom, CA.

Humphrey, S. (2003). *The Nursing Mother's Herbal*. Fairview Press.

Kennedy, D. A. (n.d.). Kennedy DA, LupattelliA, KorenG, NordengH. Safety classification of herbal medicines used in pregnancy in a multinational study. *BMC Complement Altern Med*. 2016 Mar 15;16:102. https://doi.org/10.1186/s12906-016-1079-z

Kennedy, D. A., Lupattelli, A., Koren, G., & Nordeng, H. (2013). Herbal Medicine use in pregnancy results of a multinational study. *BMC Complementary and Alternative Medicine, 13*, 355. Retrieved from https://www.scirp.org/(S(351jmbntv-nsjt1aadkposzje))/reference/referencespapers.aspx?referenceid=2757088

Khojastehfard, Z., Yazdimoghaddam, H., Abdollahi, M., & Karimi, F. (2021). Effect of Herbal Medicines on Postpartum Hemorrhage: A Systematic Review and Meta-Analysis. *Evidence Based Care, 11*(1), 62–74. https://doi.org/10.22038/ebcj.2021.58054.2513

Kloss, J. (1975). *Back to Eden: American Herbs for Pleasure and Health: Natural Nutrition with Recipes and Instruction for Living the Edenic Life.*

Louik, C., Gardiner, P., Kelley, K., & Mitchell, A. A. (2010, May). Use of herbal treatments in pregnancy. *American Journal of Obstetrics and Gynecology.* Retrieved September 8, 2022, from https://www.ncbi.nlm.nih.gov/pmc/articles/PMC2867842/

Marcian, M. (2013, July 9). Alkaloids. *The Naturopathic Herbalist.* Retrieved September 7, 2022, from https://thenaturopathicherbalist.com/plant-constituents/alkaloids/

Matsumoto, K., Horie, S., Ishikawa, H., et al. (2004). Antinociceptive effect of 7-hydroxymitragynine in mice: Discovery of an orally active opioid analgesic from the Thai medicinal herb *Mitragyna speciosa. Life Sciences, 74*, 2143–2155.

McWhirter, L., & Morris, S. (2010). A case report of inpatient detoxification after kratom (*Mitragyna speciosa*) dependence. *European Addiction Research, 16*, 229–231.

Mowrey, D. B. 1986. The scientific validation of herbal medicine. Keats Publ. New Canaan, CT.

Murray, M. T. 1995. The healing power of herbs: the enlightened person's guide to the wonders of medicinal plants. Second edition. Prima Publ. Rocklin, CA.

Pendersen, M. (1991). *Nutritional Herbology.* Pendersen Press.

Prozialeck, W. C., Jivan, J. K., & Andurkar, S. V. (2012). Pharmacology of kratom: An emerging botanical agent with stimulant, analgesic, and opioid-like effects. *The Journal of the American Osteopathic Association, 112*(12), 792–799.

Romm, A. (2010). *Botanical Medicine for Women's Health.* Churchill Livingstone.

Romm, A. J. (2014). *The Natural Pregnancy Book: Your Complete Guide to a Safe, Organic Pregnancy and Childbirth with Herbs, Nutrition, and Other Holistic Choices.* Ten Speed Press.

Sabetghadam, A., Ramanathan, S., & Mansor, S. M. (2010). The evaluation of antinociceptive activity of alkaloid, methanolic, and aqueous extracts of *Mitragyna speciosa* Korth leaves in rats. *Pharmacognosy Research, 2*(3), 181–185.

Susun Weed. (1986). *Wise Woman Herbal for the Childbearing Year.* Ash Tree Publishing.

Terzioglu Bebitoglu, B. (2020). Frequently used herbal teas during pregnancy - Short update. *Medeni Med J, 35*(1), 55–61. https://doi.org/10.5222/MMJ.2020.69851

Vicknasingam, B., Narayanan, S., Beng, G. T., & Mansor, S. M. (2010). The informal use of ketum (*Mitragyna speciosa*) for opioid withdrawal in the northern states of peninsular Malaysia and implications for drug substitution therapy. *International Journal of Drug Policy, 21*, 283–288.

Ward, J., Rosenbaum, C., Hernon, C., McCurdy, C. R., & Boyer, E. W. (2011). Herbal medicines for the management of opioid addiction. *CNS Drugs, 25*(12), 999–1007.

Weed, S. S. (1996). *Wise Woman Herbal, Healing Wise.* Ashtree Publishing.

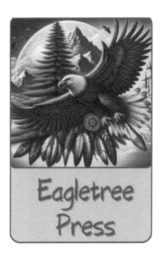